CANCER ETIOLOGY, DIAGNOSIS AND TREATMENTS

CANCEROUS TUMOR LIFE

BIOLOGICAL AND PHYSICAL ASPECTS

CANCER ETIOLOGY, DIAGNOSIS AND TREATMENTS

Additional books in this series can be found on Nova's website under the Series tab.

Additional e-books in this series can be found on Nova's website under the e-book tab.

CANCER ETIOLOGY, DIAGNOSIS AND TREATMENTS

CANCEROUS TUMOR LIFE

BIOLOGICAL AND PHYSICAL ASPECTS

MIROSŁAW KOZŁOWSKI
AND
SULTAN TARLACI

New York

For permission to use material from this book please contact us:
Telephone 631-231-7269; Fax 631-231-8175
Web Site: http://www.novapublishers.com

Additional color graphics may be available in the e-book version of this book.

Library of Congress Cataloging-in-Publication Data

ISBN: 978-1-62081-411-6

Library of Congress Control Number: 2013938080

Published by Nova Science Publishers, Inc. † New York

Contents

Preface

What is Cancer? In their seminal paper, Davies and Lineweaver (2011) developed a new theory of cancerous tumors. Until now, most research has focused on cancer as a human disease, but tumors are also widespread among animals and plants, suggesting that they have deep evolutionary roots. Indeed, cancer is such a formidable adversary because it is a fundamental part of the story of life itself. About 600 million years ago, there appeared a riot of modern-looking metazoan (the multi-celled creatures that make up the bulk of the animal kingdom), with many specialized cell types and organisms. But this explosion did not happen in a vacuum; hundreds of millions of years before, there were precursors: clumps of semi-organized cells forming robust tumor-like forms. As Davies and Lineweaver emphasized, cancer like aging must be accepted as a part of life.

In this monograph, the mutual interactions between cancer and the host body are studied. The point of view that these interactions are mediated by human consciousness is presented. The monograph consists of six chapters. Chapter 1, "Overview of the research," presents the contemporary status of the relationship between cancer and consciousness. Chapter 2, "Quantum mechanics and life," explains how quantum mechanics helps in understanding life phenomena, including cancer. Chapter 3, "Stress and cancer life," is devoted to the presentation of the possible root of cancer, namely stress, which dominates human life. Although the term 'cancer' refers to undisciplined and uncontrollable cellular growth, a basal cell carcinoma of the skin is quite different from adenocarcinoma of the lung, the prostate, the breast, or even of brain tumors, lymphomas, leukaemias and other malignancies. These all differ markedly with respect to growth rates, metastatic tendencies, and sensitivity to neuroendocrine or immune system influences, particularly those that might be modulated by stress. There are critical concerns in determining exactly how long a cancer has been present. If a lump in the breast is found to be malignant, when did the cancer start? Was it there a month, six months, or years before clinical detection? Such information would be crucial in establishing any temporal relationship with antecedent.

The remaining three chapters have a more technical character, and are devoted to the presentation of new results from the investigation of the nature of cancer. Chapter 4, "The electrical properties of cancer tumor cells," presents results concerning the physical properties of tumor cells. Chapter 5, "Classical description of tumor life: Boltzmann equation for tumor cancer evolution," presents the approach that treats cancer as a physical object. The new Boltzmann transport equation for tumor cell movement in the host body is formulated and solved. In this way, light is shed and inroads are made into answering the questions posed in Chapter 3 and beyond. Chapter 6, "Quantum mechanics and cancer," presents the quantum theory of brain waves and their possible influence on cancer proliferation. Electroencephalogram (EEG) waves may reflect more than the noise of the machinery of the brain; they may possibly represent signals being sent to other parts of the body. Since it is possible to move a cursor on a computer screen solely through deep concentration, it does not seem unreasonable to postulate that mental activities could also affect activities in the body that are sensitive to the chemical/molecular concept of communication at a physical/atomic model. Such a paradigm might explain not only regression or spontaneous remission of cancer in patients with a strong level of natural determination, but also the placebo effect, faith healing, 'therapeutic touch,' psychokinesis, telepathy, and other widely acknowledged but poorly understood concepts. How can one explain the numerous well-documented cases of spontaneous remission of cancer? Careful studies of such patients suggest that a firm faith and a strong positive belief system are the most common themes. There are numerous reports of cancer regression through the use of various stress-reducing or mind-altering techniques, including intense meditation, visual imagery, and hypnosis. Yet, like spontaneous remission, all of these cures are extremely rare, and the benefits are entirely unpredictable in any given patient. Here again, having a strong faith in something would provide a sense of control and might offer the best explanation. But how are the salutary rewards of faith healing, 'therapeutic touch,' and the placebo effect mediated? Is there such a thing as psychic healing? How can one explain the well-documented benefits associated with the development of strong social support in patients with cancer and other illnesses? Conversely, what are the mechanisms involved in the numerous reports of reactivation of dormant cancer following an extremely stressful event, particularly sudden loss? No consistent immune, neuroendocrine, or central nervous system (CNS) changes have been demonstrated in connection with such effects. Could the answer lie in some latent energy force? Adey (1992) reported that certain frequency bands between 15 and 60 Hz have been found to alter cell protein synthesis, mRNA functions, immune responses, and intercellular communication. Is it possible to learn how to harness this energy force?

Chapter I

Overview of the Research

All chemistry, including biochemistry, is based on quantum interactions. So, living systems—like non-living systems—depend on quantum states at the level of chemical bonds. However, the unitary oneness and ineffability of living systems suggest that higher level quantum properties, such as Bose-Einstein condensation, quantum coherent superposition, and entanglement, may operate in biology (Scrodinger 1994). Quantum effects are apparently washed out at scales larger than individual atoms or sub-atomic particles, at warm temperatures, and in aqueous media. Thus, the possibility of quantum states playing functional roles at mesoscopic or macroscopic scales in "warm, wet, and noisy" biological systems seems unlikely due to environmental decoherence. On the other hand, evolution may have solved the decoherence problem so that mesoscopic/macroscopic quantum states are essential features of biological systems (Hagan 2002). Living cells are 80% water, and many polar, water soluble biomolecules play key roles in cellular function. There are also extensive non-polar "oily" regions in living cells which repel water. These are called hydrophobic regions, and they occur within proteins (Hameroff 1998), lipid membranes, and nucleic acids (e.g. the "pi stack" of DNA).

If organized quantum states exist in cells, they are presumably integrated among hydrophobic regions of various cellular components and organelles. However, only proteins and geometric arrays of proteins (i.e. protein assemblies) in cytoplasm, the bulk protoplasm between cell membrane and nucleus, are considered. Proteins are folded chains of amino acids strung together by peptide bonds while the different amino acids which comprise proteins have distinct side groups with varying degrees of polarity and water solubility. Amino acids with side groups (or "residues"), which are non-polar and insoluble in water ("hydrophobic"), include phenylalanine, leucine, isoleucine, tryptophan, tyrosine, valine, and histidine (in decreasing order of hydrophobicity). The side groups in phenylalanine, tryptophan, and tyrosine ("aromatic" amino acids) are benzene-like (or "indole," in the case of tryptophan) carbon ring structures with resonant electron orbitals. (Histidine has a five sided ring with three carbons and two nitrogens.) The side groups in leucine, isoleucine, and valine have several methyl groups, each of which is a carbon with three hydrogens. Both aromatic and methyl groups are non-polar, but have electron clouds of shared, delocalizable electrons and are thus "polarizable" – dipoles can be induced in the electron clouds. The non-hydrophobic amino acids have side groups which are charged, or polar, and thus soluble in water (Voet 1995). As proteins fold into their functional shapes, hydrophobic groups avoid the liquid environment and bury themselves together in the protein interior, forming hydrophobic pockets, not unlike oil droplets forming in, or on the surface of, water. It is, in fact, the hydrophobic effect and attractions among non-polar hydrophobic groups by van der Waals forces which drive protein folding. Although the confluence of hydrophobic side groups is small – roughly 1/30 to 1/250 of protein volumes – it exerts enormous influence in the regulation of protein dynamics and function. (Several hydrophobic pockets may work cooperatively in a single protein.) Hydrophobic pockets may be considered the "brain" or nervous system of each protein. Proteins change shape over a number of time scales (Karplus 1983). Small parts of proteins, for example, protrusions from the main body of the protein, change as fast as femtoseconds (10^{-15} sec). Other conformational changes are very slow. The binding of oxygen by blood hemoglobin changes the shape of hemoglobin until the oxygen is released, a process that may take many seconds or minutes. Most functional conformational transitions in which the entire protein globally changes shape occur in the time scale of nanoseconds (10^{-9} sec) to 10 picoseconds (10^{-11} sec). An ion channel, for example, may change its shape in a nanosecond or so, but remain open long enough for ions to flow through. Interactions among side groups within proteins provide a large amount of energy, e.g. thousands of kilojoules per mole (kJ mol^{-1}). Yet proteins are only marginally stable against denaturation by an excess of 40 kJ mol^{-1}, while switching and conformational changes in proteins may be triggered by very small amounts of energy. For example, open and closed states of the potassium channel differ by only small amounts of energy, regulated by a hydrophobic lever (Jiang 2003).

How do such high energy systems change shape due to extremely low energy stimuli? The answer seems to be that high energy interactions from chemical and ionic bonding among charged, polar side groups tend to cancel out, such that protein conformation is a "delicate balance among powerful countervailing forces" (Voet 1995). More dynamic, low energy interactions such as the forces active in non-polar hydrophobic pockets are thus leveraged or amplified to regulate conformation. These are the van der Waals forces. Additionally, London forces have important biological implications. Anesthetic gases act to ablate consciousness in hydrophobic pockets of certain brain proteins (Hameroff 1995). The anesthetic gas molecules do so by forming their own van der Waals London interactions with non-polar amino acid groups in the pockets. This, presumably, impairs normally occurring London force effects which are necessary for protein functions that are required for consciousness. How are movements of electrons, even collective movements of many electrons, able to tip the "delicate balance of countervailing forces" in proteins in order to cause conformational changes in the range of nanoseconds to ten picoseconds? Due to the Mossbauer Effect, electronic motions should couple to nuclear motions (and thus conformation) via a recoil phenomenon (Hameroff & Tuszynski 2003). However, the nuclear/conformational movement would be slight. Because of the small mass of electrons relative to that of protons and neutrons, a one nanometer shift of a single electron would move the nuclear mass, and hence protein conformation by only 10^{-8} nanometers, the diameter of a single carbon atom nucleus. However, the charge of each electron is equivalent to that of protons, and collective electron charge movements by London forces are thus able to influence nuclear motion and protein conformation (Conrad 1994). London forces are quantum effects; the instantaneous dipoles are actually probabilistic densities of electron clouds. If the electron dipoles couple to protein conformation, then proteins should exist in quantum superposition of different conformations, albeit of very small separations. For example, the Mossbauer shift of 10^{-8} nanometers would mean that the protein's nuclei, and thus the protein, would separate "from itself" by this distance – the diameter of a carbon atom nucleus. But even this slight separation, coupled cooperatively among atomic nuclei throughout the protein, may tip "the balance between countervailing forces." So a protein in superposition of two locations which differ by 10^{-8} nanometers may collapse/reduce/decohere into two distinct conformations which differ in location from each other by several angstroms. Proteins may then be considered to act as quantum bits, or "qubits."

Some evidence supports quantum effects in hydrophobic pockets playing functional roles in determining protein conformation. Roitberg (1995) showed functional protein vibrations which depend on quantum effects centered in two hydrophobic phenylalanine side groups, and Tejada, et al. (1996) have evidence to suggest quantum coherent states exist in the protein ferritin. Nonlocal quantum interactions (Klein-Seetharaman 2002) and quantum tunneling appear to guide protein folding (Satinover 2001). Such effects are confined to individual proteins, and the role of the environment must be considered. Polar amino acid side groups which interface with the protein's external milieu may allow environmental effects to dominate, relegating the protein to a "slave." Random thermal motion in an aqueous environment would promote decoherence and prevent or disrupt quantum states. However structured, cooperative environments may allow collective effects promoting the large scale quantum coherence of proteins. Living material is termed 'protoplasm,' which includes cell membranes and cell interiors. Cell interiors, excluding the nucleus, are comprised of organelles embedded in cytoplasm, which is composed mainly of water and networks/matrices of proteins collectively termed the cytoskeleton. There are three main components of the cytoskeleton: actin, intermediate filaments, and microtubules, all organized around a central focus called the centrosome. Situated just outside and adjacent to the cell nucleus, the centrosome is composed of a curious organelle called the centriole, which is embedded in an electron-rich protein medium.

Actin protein is the most dynamic cytoskeletal structure, rapidly polymerizing and depolymerizing, and, by doing so, changing the character of cytoplasm from a liquid phase ("sol," i.e. solution) when actin is disassembled, to a solid gelatinous phase ("gel") when actin is assembled/polymerized (Pollack 2001). Such "sol-gel transitions," which can occur as rapidly as 40 times per second, account for intracellular flow of cytoplasm (e.g. "amoeboid movement"). Because actin surfaces are negatively charged in the gel phase, nearly all polar cell water molecules are bound and "ordered." Thus, during the gel phase, the view of cell interiors as a "minestrone soup" of floating organelles is incorrect. Rather, cytoplasmic gel is a quasi-solid state medium. Intermediate filaments are fairly stable, and their precise function is poorly understood. On the other hand, microtubules can be either stable or dynamic, and play many essential roles in cell biology. In asymmetrical cells such as neurons (with long extensions called axons and dendrites), microtubules play structural roles, as more or less permanent girders. During cell division, or "mitosis," microtubules depolymerize and then repolymerize as mitotic spindles, separating "daughter chromosomes" and establishing the architecture for daughter cells. The microtubule spindles pull the daughter chromosomes toward two poles anchored by centrioles which seem to guide navigation and cytoplasmic organization. Each centriole is a pair of barrel-like structures arranged curiously in perpendicular tandem, and (like mitotic spindles) are comprised of microtubules There are a number of issues regarding mitosis, but one compelling question is how the processes are coordinated in space and time by centrioles in order to generate a geometric spindle structure that maintains itself at steady state. A review in *Science* concluded: "Robustness of spindle assembly must come from guidance of microtubules by a field (Karesenti 2001). Microtubules are cylindrical polymers of the protein tubulin and are 25 nanometers (nm) in diameter (Dustin 1984). The cylinder walls of microtubules are comprised of 13 longitudinal protofilaments which are each a series of tubulin subunits. Each tubulin subunit is an 8 nm by 4 nm by 5 nm heterodimer which consists of two slightly different classes of 4 nm, 55,000 dalton monomers known as alpha and beta tubulin. The tubulin dimer subunits within the cylinder walls are arranged in a hexagonal lattice which is slightly twisted, resulting in differing neighbor relationships among each subunit and its six nearest neighbors. Pathways along neighbor tubulins form helices which repeat on any protofilament every 3, 5, 8, 13, etc. rows (the "Fibonacci series").

Each tubulin has a surplus of negative surface charges, with a majority on the alpha monomer; thus, each tubulin is a permanent dipole (beta plus, alpha minus). Consequently, microtubules can be considered "electrets": oriented assemblies of dipoles which are predicted to have piezoelectric, ferroelectric, and spin glass properties (Tuszyński 1995). In addition, negatively charged C–termini "tails" extend outward from each monomer, attracting positive ions from the cytoplasm and forming a plasma-like "Debye layer" surrounding the microtubule (Hameroff 2003). Biochemical energy is provided to microtubules in several ways: tubulin-bound GTP is hydrolyzed to GDP in microtubules, and microtubule associated proteins which attach at specific points on the microtubule lattice are phosphorylated. In addition, microtubules may possibly utilize nonspecific thermal energy for "laser-like" coherent pumping, for example, in the GigaHz range by a mechanism of "pumped phonons" suggested by Fröhlich (Fröhlich 1968, 1970, 1975). Simulations of coherent phonons in microtubules suggest that phonon maxima correspond with functional binding sites of microtubule associated proteins (Samsonowich 1992). In centrioles (as well as cilia, flagella, basal bodies, etc.) microtubules fuse into doublets or triplets. Nine doublets or triplets then form larger barrel-like cylinders which, in some cases, have internal structures connecting the doublets/triplets. Two cylinders in perpendicular tandem form the centriole which initiates and organizes mitosis (cell division) and other cell movements. Centrioles and cilia are involved in photoreceptor functions in single cell organisms and primitive visual systems (Albrech-Buehler 1992). Cilia are also found in all retinal rod and cone cells. The dimensions of centrioles and cilia are equivalent to wavelengths of visible and infrared light, and waveguide functions have been suggested. Because mitosis (cell division) is organized by centrioles and requires precise, mirror-like activities, quantum entanglement mediated by quantum optical effects between centrioles has been proposed (Hameroff 2004). To account for communication and organization in living systems, physicists (Fröhlich 1975) have suggested that a membrane or large chain of macromolecules possessing longitudinal dipole vibrations could act like a Bose-Einstein condensate. Fröhlich's proposal was based on the notion that biological systems are far from equilibrium, and have considerable amounts of available energy which lead to non-linear behaviors. The concept that body systems not in equilibrium and governed by nonlinear kinetic laws may display macroscopic self-organized order is consistent with approaches such as Prigogine's dissipative structures and Haken's synergetics.

In Fröhlich's model, several modes of dipole vibrations are excited by a continuous supply of metabolic energy. The electric vibrations couple with acoustic vibrations inherent in the structure through non-linear dynamics; Fröhlich specified dipoles in hydrophobic regions of proteins as the relevant dipoles in this process. If the supplied energy is sufficiently large relative to the energy lost, the system attains a stationary state in which the dipole vibrations channel into a single longitudinal mode (the one with minimum frequency). The common mode increases its population enormously in a way reminiscent of Bose-Einstein condensation. The single mode, which can exhibit long range correlations, is thus akin to laser-like coherent pumped phonons in the range of 10^9 to 10^{11} Hz. The proposed frequency is in the microwave range (Grundler 1983) and corresponds to recognized protein conformational transitions in the range of nanoseconds to 10 picoseconds. Fröhlich's proposal may be seen in a context of quantum field theory whose proponents have viewed living matter as a sea of electric dipoles organized by electret states, and the consequent ordering of water around biomolecules, providing collective states of ordered symmetry (Pessa 2001).

In a typical *non-biological* system, component dipoles are random and disordered, resulting in an overall symmetry ("rotationally invariant"). In living systems, order is induced by rotational alignment along filamentous electrets such as microtubules and other cytoskeletal structures. According to quantum field theory and the "Goldstone theorem," symmetry breaking ("Bose condensation") results in long range interactions among system components (dipoles) conveyed by massless particle/waves ("Goldstone bosons"). The energy required to generate massless bosons is invested in the electret states of biomolecules and correlated fluctuations in their surrounding water and ions. For example, Celashi and Mascarenhas (Celaschi, Mascarenhas, 1977) showed that electret activation energy of biomolecules (0.2–0.4 electron volts) is equivalent to the hydrolysis of one ATP or GTP molecule and what Davydov predicted for initiation of solitons (Hall 1996). Consequently, solitons, massless bosons, and Fröhlich's coherent polarization waves may be synonymous. Del Giudice (1982, 1983) concluded that electromagnetic energy penetrating into cytoplasm would be confined *inside filaments* whose diameters depended on the original symmetry breaking ("Bose condensation") of ordered dipoles. Any electric disturbance produced by thermally fluctuating dipoles, or by any other source, would be confined inside filamentous regions. Ordering is preserved outside the filaments and is disrupted only inside where energy becomes concentrated (the "Meissner effect"). The diameter of the self-focusing energy filaments depends on the polarization density, or ordering of biological water. Del Guidice's group calculated a self-focusing diameter of about 15 nanometers, which is *precisely the inner diameter of a microtubule*, and concluded that the cytoskeleton is the material consequence of dynamic self-focusing of polarization waves in the cytoplasm. The observed diameters of self-focused optical beams in simple *non-biological* liquids are of the order of microns; correlation among components is created by propagation of waves rather than as a specific property of the material itself. Thus, focusing occurs in cytoplasm of eukaryotic cells due to the spatial coherence and ordering imparted by cytoskeletal electret behavior. Along similar lines, Jibu and Yasue (1994, 1995) calculated that Fröhlich dynamics of ordered water on microtubule surfaces, particularly the internal hollow core of microtubules, would result in quantum optical modes termed super-radiance and self-induced transparency. Evanescent quantum photons in the infra-red region would propagate without loss, in an optical analogue to superconductivity. The quantum coherent state would involve a region of 50 microns, allowing quantum coherence to spread through tissues.

Another relevant approach is through the zero point energy of the quantum vacuum. Virtual particle/waves (photons) in the quantum vacuum "pop into and out of existence," giving rise to a description of spacetime as the "quantum foam." Zero point energy may be measured through the Casimir effect. For example, two parallel plates can be held closely together such that the narrow gap excludes photons whose wavelength is larger than the gap. The relative surplus of photons outside of the gap exerts a force pushing the plates together. Experiments with parallel plates placed 0.6 to 6.0 microns apart confirm the Casimir effect, finding a very small, but measurable force pushing the plates together. Lamoreux (1997) and Hall (1996) calculated the Casimir force on a microtubule whose cavity diameter ("*d*") is 15 nanometers, roughly 100 times smaller than the gap *d* in the described experiment. As the force depends on d^{-4}, the Casimir effect would be a million times greater (neglecting effects of the cylindrical surface compared to the planar surface). Depending on length, Hall calculated a Casimir pressure of 0.5 to 20 atmospheres on a microtubule. In a specific proposal for a mechanism of consciousness, Penrose and Hameroff (1998) have suggested that microtubules function as quantum computers, with tubulin proteins within microtubules acting as quantum bits, or qubits. The model (Orchestrated objective reduction, Orch OR) is summarized as follows: conformational states of individual tubulins within neuronal microtubules are determined by quantum mechanical London forces within the tubulin interiors which can induce conformational quantum superposition.

While in superposition, tubulins communicate/compute with entangled tubulins in the same microtubule, in other microtubules in the same neuron, in microtubules in neighboring neurons, and through macroscopic regions of the brain by tunneling through gap junctions and possibly tunneling through nanotubes. Quantum states of tubulin/microtubules are isolated/protected from environmental decoherence by biological mechanisms which include phases of actin gelation, ordered water, plasma-like Debye layering, coherent pumping and topological quantum error correction. Microtubule quantum computations/superpositions are tuned or 'orchestrated' by microtubule associated proteins during a classical, liquid phase which alternates (e.g., at 40 Hz) with a quantum, solid state phase of actin gelation. Following periods of pre-conscious quantum computation (e.g., in the order of tens to hundreds of milliseconds) tubulin superpositions reduce or collapse by Penrose quantum gravity 'objective reduction' (OR). The classical output states, which result from the OR process, are chosen non-algorithmically ('non-computably') and govern neural events by binding microtubule-associated proteins, regulating synapses and membrane functions, etc. The reduction or 'self-collapse' in the orchestrated objective reduction 'Orch OR' model is suggested to be a 'conscious moment,' linked to Penrose's quantum gravity mechanism which ties the process to fundamental spacetime geometry. This connection enables a panprotopsychist approach to the 'hard problem' of subjective experience. This implies that tubulins can exist in quantum superposition of two or more possible states until the threshold for quantum state reduction (i.e., by Penrose quantum gravity mediated "objective reduction") is reached. The tubulin superposition is suggested to involve separation of tubulin "from itself" by a Fermi length, which is the diameter of an atomic (i.e., carbon) nucleus. Despite the slight separation distance, the two states presumably evolve to functional conformations which differ in location by angstroms. Not surprisingly, the Penrose-Hameroff Orch OR model has engendered criticism because of the apparent and obvious problem of decoherence.

Cytoplasm is considered to be a hostile environment for mesoscopic or macroscopic quantum states because it is viewed as "warm, wet, and noisy," all of which would presumably lead to decoherence of quantum states. Consider these objections: *"Warm"* – quantum information technologies are constructed at absolute zero temperatures to avoid thermal decoherence. By those standards, biological systems are sizzling hot. For example, humans function at around 37.6 degrees centigrade. However, some quantum states, like lasers, do function at warm temperatures, and are energetically pumped to produce quantum coherence. In the Fröhlich approach, thermal energy is used in a similar fashion to pump coherence in lattices of dipoles. Microtubules and other cytoskeletal lattice structures are ideal for such a mechanism. Moreover, quantum spin transfer between quantum dots connected by benzene rings (the same structures found in aromatic hydrophobic amino acids) is more efficient at warm temperatures than at absolute zero (Ouyang 2003). The authors hypothesize that the "flexibility" of the resonant benzene electrons is advantageous to quantum processes by harnessing ambient thermal energy. *"Wet"* – cytoplasm is often viewed as an aqueous medium in virtue of its water content of 80%. Yet, when actin is polymerized, cell water is apparently completely ordered resulting in a quasi-solid state medium (Pollack 2001). Moreover, ordered water at cytoskeletal surfaces would also be driven by Fröhlich coherence pumped by heat and biochemical energy. The sum total of hydrophobic space in interiors of proteins, membranes, and nucleic acids provides a non-polar, spatially-distributed region throughout living systems.

"*Noisy.*" it is assumed that the aqueous, thermal cytoplasmic environment is noisy. However, if coherent pumping and ordered water occur, noise may not be an issue. In the brain, apparent noise in terms of electrically-recorded membrane fluctuations have been found to have long range correlations, and thus may not be noise, but rather some underlying coupling. Attempting to disprove the possibility of quantum computation in brain microtubules, University of Pennsylvania physicist Tegmark (2000) calculated that microtubule quantum states at physiological temperatures would decohere a trillion times too fast for physiological effects, with a calculated decoherence time of 10^{-13} seconds. Neurons generally function in the range of roughly 10 to 100 milliseconds, or 10^{-2} to 10^{-1} seconds. Tegmark did not actually address specifics of the Penrose-Hameroff Orch OR model, nor any previous theory, but rather proposed his own quantum microtubule model which he did successfully disprove. For example, Tegmark assumed quantum superposition of a soliton wave traveling along a microtubule, "separated from itself" by 24 nanometers. The Penrose-Hameroff model actually proposed quantum superposition of tubulin proteins separated from themselves by the diameter of their atomic nuclei. This discrepancy alone accounts for a difference of seven orders of magnitude in the decoherence calculation. Moreover, Tegmark did not consider other factors included in the Penrose-Hameroff proposal such as plasma phase screening, actin gel isolation, coherent pumping, and quantum error correction topology intrinsic to microtubule geometry (Hagan, Tegmark 2002). Tegmark's own decoherence formula, and correcting for the stipulations in the Penrose-Hameroff model, calculated microtubule decoherence times in the range of 10^{-2} to 10^{-1} seconds or longer (without benefit of topological quantum error correction).

Technological quantum computation became more feasible with the advent of quantum error correction codes in the early 1990s (Steane 1992). This means that algorithms run on a quantum computer can detect and correct errors due to random localized decoherence before they destroy the global quantum state. In some cases, specific topological structural geometry of the quantum computer enhances the error correction. For example, toroidal surfaces may have global, topological degrees of freedom which are protected from local errors and decoherence (Freedman 2002). The topology of microtubule lattices involves helical windings which repeat on any given protofilament according to the Fibonacci series (3, 5, 8, 13, 21…). Each of the winding patterns also corresponds with pathways along specific aromatic amino acid groups which may promote exciton or spin transfer along those pathways (Hameroff 2002). If in the winding patterns, subunits are taken as qubits rather than individual tubulin, then microtubules may be resistant to decoherence by virtue of topological quantum error correction. If any individual tubulin in a winding decoheres, it will resonate back into quantum superposition by other tubulins. In this scenario, the output of the quantum computation will be specific combinations of winding patterns which are known to induce binding of microtubule-associated proteins which in turn determine cytoskeletal structure and function. This may also be seen to utilize the Aharonov-Bohm effect in which alternate loop pathways may exist in quantum superposition. Recent quantum information technology utilizes unpaired electron quantum spin (rather than electron location) to represent information ("spintronics").

As previously mentioned, electron quantum spin transfer through organic benzene molecules (the same as found in aromatic amino acids) is more efficient at room temperature than at absolute zero (Ouyang 2003). At physiological temperature, unpaired electron spins form networks in protein interiors (Binihi, 2002), and nonlocal quantum effects are important in protein folding. What about microtubules and spintronics? Microtubules are ferromagnetic lattices which align parallel to strong magnetic fields, which may be accounted for by single unpaired electrons per tubulin. Atomic structure of a tubulin shows two positively charged areas (~100-150 meV) near the alpha-beta dimer "neck," separated by a negatively charged area of about 1.5 nanometers. This negatively-charged region constitutes a double well potential which should enable inter-well quantum tunneling of single electrons and spin states since the energy depth is significantly above thermal fluctuations (kT=25 meV at room temperature). The intra-tubulin dielectric constant is only 2, compared to roughly 80 outside the microtubule. Hence, neither environmental nor thermal effects threaten quantum spin states in the double well. A number of possible implementations of organized quantum states and processes in cytoplasm have been discussed, suggesting that such states and processes are relevant to the essential features of living systems.

What *is* life? Life is a process generally described in terms of its properties and functions such as self-organization, metabolism (energy utilization), adaptive behavior, reproduction, and evolution. Whether or not this functional description is complete is a matter of contention. Two broad types of approaches have attempted to characterize the essential nature of the life process: (1) functionalism and (2) vitalism.

Functionalism implies that life is independent of its material substrate. For example, certain types of self-organizing computer programs can exhibit life-like functions, and "artificial life" proponents view such systems as "alive." Functionalists also point out that life's material substrate does not distinguish biological matter. Proteins, DNA, carbohydrates, fats, and other biomolecular components are made of the same atoms and elements that make up inanimate substances. Bolstered by the success of genetic engineering, functional/reductive approaches dominate molecular biology. "Life" is ascribed to an emergent property of biochemical processes. Nonetheless, a commonly held contrary viewpoint is that functional descriptions fail to capture an essential self- organizing "unitary oneness" present in living systems. To nineteenth-century biologists, this quality was ascribed to a "life force," "*elan vital*," or energy field. Then, as molecular and cell biology began to reveal the biochemical and physical processes involved in cellular activities, the apparent need for a life force waned, and "vitalists" (or "animists") were vilified. In modern reductionist science, the notion of a life force, energy, or information field has remained almost taboo. However, nineteenth-century vitalism was based either completely on electromagnetism or on forces outside the realm of science. Quantum effects were unknown.

There are three types of theories regarding the origin of life. One involves a Creator, the second involves spontaneous chemical activity leading to biomolecules, and the third involves seeding of the earth from extraterrestrial sources. The extraterrestrial theory (e.g., life carried by meteorites) is supported by the timing of life's evolutionary development on earth, but still requires an explanation for life's origin somewhere else (Line 2002). Peptides, simple sugars, lipids, and nucleic acid could have formed spontaneously in salt water in tide pools, near thermal vents, or in clay minerals (Cairus-Smith 1986). The big mystery is how these simple biomolecular precursors evolved to organelles and cells. Proteins, lipids, and nucleic acids are composed of constituent molecules which have both non-polar and polar regions on opposite ends. In an aqueous medium, the non-polar regions of any of these components will join together to form hydrophobic regions where quantum forces reign. Perhaps the first forms of life were tiny oil-like pockets—shielded from the aqueous environment—in which quantum interactions organized, linked together, and regulated increasingly larger biomolecules. As non-polar aromatic groups absorb and are excited by photons, organized arrays of such groups (i.e., cytoskeletal structures) may have induced cytoplasm to evolve as phase-ordered matter (Scully 2003). In cytoplasm, cytoskeletal structures and ordered water on their surfaces are ideal media for quantum coherence. As suggested by Fröhlich, these structures would be able to utilize nonspecific metabolic energy and heat to promote coherence (rather than decoherence), and possibly generate, perceive, and trap evanescent photons. The evolutionary origin of centrioles, cilia, and flagella (which have the same basic structure of nine microtubule doublets or triplets arranged in a larger cylinder, but with additional motor proteins) is unclear. According to endosymbiotic theory (Margulis 1975), eukaryotic cells arose from symbiosis, an invasion of simple bacteria-like prokaryotes by mitochondria which supplied energy, and by flagellates (e.g., spirochetes) which brought cytoskeletal proteins providing structural support, compartmentalization, internal organization, movement, perhaps intelligence, and eventually consciousness. The origin of flagellates is unknown. There is some question as to whether centrioles, cilia, and flagella (i.e., flagellates) could have evolved purely by natural selection, as they are said to exhibit "irreducible complexity" (White 2000).

References

Albrecht–Buehler A, 1992, *Rudimentary form of cellular "vision"* , Proc. Natl Acad Sci, USA, 89(17), 8288-8292.

Bairoch A, Apweiler R, 1998, *The swiss-prot protein sequence data bank and its supplement TrEMBL*, Nucl. Acids Res., 26, 38-42.

Binhi V N, Savin A V, 2002, *Molecular gyroscopes and biological effects of weak extremely low-frequency magnetic fields*, Phys Rev E, 65: 051912-1&8211:051912-1.

Cairns-Smith A G, 1986, Clay Minerals and the Origin of Life, Cambridge University Press, Cambridge.

Celaschi S, Mascarenhas S, 1977, *Thermal stimulated pressure and current studies of bound water in lysozyme*, Biophys. J., 29(2), 273-277.

Conrad M, 1994, *Amplification of superpositional effects through electronic conformational interactions,* Chaos, Solitons and Fractals, 4, 423-438.

Davies P C W, 2001, *Physics and life, in the first steps of life in the Universe*, Proceedings of the Sixth Trieste Conference on Chemical Evolution, Editors: J. Chela-Flores, Owen, Tobias, F. Raulin, Academic Publishers, Dordrecht, The Netherlands, 18-22 September.

Del Giudice E, et al., 1983,*Spontaneous symmetry breakdown and boson condensation in Biology,* Phys. Rev. Letts, 95(a), 508–51.

Del Giudice E, et al., 1982, *Self focusing of Fröhlich Waves and Cytoskeleton Dynamics*, Phys. Letts, 90A, 104–106.

Del Giudice E, 1986, Collective Properties of Biological Systems In: Modern Bioelectrochemistry. F. Gutmann and H. Keyzer eds, Plenum Press, New York.

Dustin P, 1984, Microtubules, 2nd Revised Ed, Springe, Berlin.

Frauenfelder H, et al., 2002, *Hydration, slaving and protein function,* Biophysical Chemistry, *98(1-2):35-48.*

Freedman A, et al., 2002, Topological quantum error correction quant-ph/0101025.

Fröhlich H, 1968, *Long-range coherence and energy storage in biological systems*, Int. J. Quantum Chem, 2, 6419.

Fröhlich H, 1970, *Long-range coherence and the actions of enzymes,* Nature, 228, 1093.

Fröhlich H, 1975, *The extraordinary dielectric properties of biological materials and the action of enzymes*, Proc. Natl. Acad. Sci, 72, 4211-4215.

Grinvald A, et al., 2003, *Neuronal assemblies: single cortical neurons are obedient members of a huge orchestra*, Biopolymers, 68(3), 422-36.

Grundler W, Keilmann F, 1983, Sharp resonances in yeast growth proved nonthermal sensitivity to microwaves. Phys. Rev. Letts, 51, 1214-1216.

Hagan Hameroff S, Tuszynski, J, 2002, *Quantum computation in brain microtubules? decoherence and biological feasibility*, Physical Reviews E, 65, 061901.

Hall G L, 1996, *Quantum electrodynamic (QED) fluctuations in various models of neuronal microtubules*, Consciousness Research Abstracts -Tucson II (Journal of Consciousness Studies), Abstract, 145.

Hameroff S, nd, *A new theory of cancer: Centrioles, mitosis and quantum entanglement*, submitted.

Hameroff S et al., nd, *Molecular automata in microtubules: basic computational logic of the living state*, Artifical Life: SFI Studies in the Science of Complexity, ed. C. Langton, Addison-Wesley, New York, pp. 521-553.

Hameroff S, Penrose R, 1996, *Orchestrated reduction of quantum coherence in brain microtubules: a model for consciousness*, eds. S.R. Hameroff, A. Kaszniak, and Scott Toward a Science of Consciousness The First Tucson Discussions and Debates, MIT Press, Cambridge, MA. Also published in: *Mathematics and Computers in Simulation*, 40, 453-480.

Hameroff S, 1998, *Quantum computation in brain microtubules? The Penrose-Hameroff 'Orch OR' model of consciousness*, Philosophical Transactions Royal Society, London (A) 356, 1869-1896.

Hameroff S, 1998, *Anesthesia, consciousness and hydrophobic pockets,* Toxicology Letters, 100/101:31-39.

Hameroff S. Penrose R, 1996, *Conscious events as orchestrated spacetime selections*, Journal of Consciousness Studies, 3(1), 36-53.

Hameroff S, Tuszynski. J, 2003, *Search for quantum and classical modes of information processing in microtubules: implications for the living state*, Bioenergetic Organization in Living Systems, eds. Franco Musumeci, Mae-Wan Ho, World Scientific, Singapore.

Hameroff S., et al., 2003, *Conduction pathways in microtubules, biological quantum computation, and consciousness*, BioSystems, 64, 149-168.

Hameroff. S, 1997, *Quantum vitalism*, Advances: The Journal of Mind-Body Health, 13(4), 13-22.

Hirokawa M, 1991, *Molecular architecture and dynamics of the neuronal cytoskeleton*, The Neuronal Cytoskeleton, ed. R. Burgoyne. New York, Wiley-Liss, pp. 5-74.

Jiang Y, Ruta V J, Chen J, Lee A, MacKinnon R, 2003, *The principle of gating charge movement in a voltage- dependent K+ channel*, Nature, 423(6935), 42-8.

Jibu M et al., 1994, *Quantum optical coherence in cytoskeletal microtubules: implications for brain function*, BioSystems, 32, 195-209.

Jibu M et al., 1994, *Quantum optical coherence in cytoskeletal microtubules: implications for brain function*, BioSystems, 32:195-209.

Jibu M, Yasue K, 1995, *Quantum brain dynamics: an introduction*. John Benjamins, Amsterdam.

Karplus M, McCammon J A, 1983, *Protein ion channels, gates, receptors*, In. Dynamics of Proteins: Elements and Function, Ann. Rev. Biochem, ed. J. King, Benjamin/Cummings, Menlo Park, 40, 263-300.

Karsenti E, Vernos I, 2001, *The mitotic spindle: A self-made machine*, Science 294, 543-547.

Klein-Seetharaman J et al., 2002, *Long-range interactions within a nonnative protein*, Science, 295, 1719-1722.

Lamoreaux S K, 1997, *Demonstration of the Casimir force in the 0.6 to 6 micron range*, Physical Review Letters, 78(1), 5-8.

Lauck L, et al., 1992, *On Fröhlich's coherent effects in biological systems: influence of carriers and high order dissipative effects*, J Theor Biol, 158, 1-13.

Line M A, 2002, *The enigma of life and its timing*?, Microbiology, 148, 21-27.

Margulis L,1975, *Origin of Eukaryotic Cells*. Yale University Press, New Haven.

Nogale E, Wolf S G, Downing K, 1998, *Structure of the tubulin dimer by electron crystallography*, Nature, 391, 199-203.

Ouyang M, Awschalom DD, *Coherent spin transfer between molecularly bridged quantum dots*, Science, 301, 1074-1078.

Penrose R, Hameroff S, 1995, *Gaps, what gaps? Reply to Grush and Churchland*, Journal of Consciousness Studies, 2(2), 99-112.

Pessa E, Vitiello G, 1999, *Quantum dissipation and neural net dynamics*, Bioelectrochemistry & Bioenergetics, 48(2), 339-42.

Pollack G. H, 2001, *Cells, Gels and the Engines of Life*, Ebner and Sons, Seattle.

Reid B L, Bourke C, 2001, *Attempts to identify a control system for chemical reactivity in the living state using virtual energy*, Medical Hypotheses, 57(1), 6-22.

Roitberg A, Gerber R B, Elber R, Ratner M, 1995, *Anharmonic wave functions of proteins: quantum self consistent field calculations of BPTI*, Science, 268(5315), 1319-1322.

Samsonovich A, et al., 1992, *Acousto-conformational transitions in cytoskeletal microtubules: Implications for information processing*, Nanobiology, 1, 457-468.

Satinover J, 2001, *The Quantum Brain*, Wiley and Sons, New York.

Schrodinger E, 1944, *What is Life?* Cambridge University Press, Cambridge UK.

Scully M O, 2003, *Light at a standstill?* Nature, 426, 610-611.

Steane A, nd, *Introduction to quantum error correction*, Phil. Trans. Roy. Soc. Lond, A, 356, 1739-1758.

Tegmark M, 2000, *The importance of quantum decoherence in brain processes*, Phys. Rev. E, 61, 4194–4206.

Tejada A, et al., 1996, *Does macroscopic quantum coherence occur in ferritin?* Science, 272, 424-426.

Tuszynski J, et al., 1995, *Ferroelectric behavior in microtubule dipole lattices; implications for information processing, signaling and assembly/disassembly*, J. Theor. Biol. 174, 371-380.

Voet D, Voet J G, 1995, *Biochemistry*, Wiley, 2nd edition, New York, 1995.

White S, et al., 2000, *Educators have a hard choice nationally, not just in Kansas*, Science, 289(5481), 869-71.

Chapter II

Quantum Mechanics and Life

Conceptualizing cancer in an evolutionary context promises to transform the understanding of the condition and offer new therapeutic possibilities (Merlo et al. 2006). Conversely, a proper understanding of cancer will inform evolutionary biology and astrobiology by casting important light on the nature and evolution of complex life and the origin of multicellularity. A longstanding criticism of cancer biology and oncological research is that it has so far taken little account of evolutionary biology (Nesse, Williams 1996). Cancer is the result of the proliferation of misregulated cells belonging to the host organism, and while the onset of some cancers may be triggered by viral infection, or chemical carcinogens, cancer itself is not an infection. Cancer cells are the cells of our own bodies, not foreign viruses or bacteria. With the possible exception of the naked mole-rat (Suluanov et al. 2009), it is likely that cancer occurs in almost all metazoans in which adult cells proliferate. This quasi-ubiquity suggests that the mechanisms of cancer are deep-rooted in evolutionary history, a hypothesis that receives support from both paleontology and genetics. Dinosaur tumors, for example, have been documented many times (Rothschild et al. 2003), and some oncogenes (genes thought to be responsible for causing cancer) are extremely ancient.

These tumors' precursors were already present in similar form in the primitive metazoans that served as common ancestors to chordates and arthropods, according to Weinberg (1983). Recent genetic studies of a freshwater Hydra indicate that the human oncogene 'myc' dates back at least 600 million years (Hartl et al. 2010), while more comprehensive studies reveal even older dates (Srivastava et al. 2010). Weinberg (1983) speculated on the implications of the fact that the genes that cause cancer are ancient and highly conserved: "Such conservation indicates that these genes have served vital, indispensable functions in normal cellular and organismic physiology, and that their role in carcinogenesis represents only an unusual and aberrant diversion from their usual functions." It has become clear that the genes responsible for the cellular cooperation necessary for multicellularity are also the genes that malfunction in cancer cells (Weinberg 2007).

In this book, we further the idea that cancer has deep evolutionary roots and make specific predictions based on the connection between cancer and the evolution of multicellularity. Our central hypothesis is that cancer is an atavistic state of multicellular life. Atavisms occur because genes for previously-existing traits are often preserved in a genome, but are switched off or relegated to non-coding ('junk') segments of DNA. For example, humans are sometimes born with tails, webbed feet, gills, hypertrichosis, and supernumerary nipples (Le Page 2007). Mutant chickens can be induced to form teeth (Gould 1980, Chen et al. 2000. Harris et al. 2006). Atavisms result from the malfunction of the more-recently-evolved genes that suppress such ancestral developments (Hall 1984, Harris et al. 2006). Hens' teeth, or cetaceans' hind legs are atavisms expressing ancestral genes that became inhibited 60 million years ago (Gould 1980, Chen et al. 2000). Traditionally, atavisms are associated with the morphological features of the developing zygote. Here, we propose that cancer is an atavism associated with ancestral cellular functions regulated by genes that have been largely suppressed for more than 600 million years. The transition from unicellular to complex multicellular organisms took place over an extended period starting at least 1 billion years ago (Hedges, Kumar 2009). Importantly, 'advanced' metazoan life of the form we now know – i.e., organisms with cell specialization and organ differentiation – was preceded by colonies of eukaryotic cells in which cellular cooperation was fairly rudimentary, consisting of networks of adhering cells exchanging information chemically, and forming self-organized assemblages with only moderate division of labor. These proto-metazoans were effectively small, loosely-knit ecosystems that fell short of the complex organization and regulation we associate with most modern metazoans. In short, proto-metazoans, which we dub Metazoans 1.0, were tumor-like neoplasms.

By 600 million years ago, Metazoa 2.0 had emerged. These organisms have a richer repertoire of biological processes needed to coordinate a larger number of highly-differentiated cell types. They are characterized by sophisticated genetic and epigenetic command and control systems familiar from modern complex organisms, such as humans. It is, however, in the nature of Darwinian evolution that life builds opportunistically on what has gone before. The genetic apparatus of the new Metazoa 2.0 was overlain on the old genetic apparatus of Metazoa 1.0. The genes of Metazoa 1.0 were tinkered with where possible, and suppressed where necessary by nature. But many of these unnecessary genes are still present, constituting a robust toolkit for the survival, maintenance, and propagation of non-differentiated or weakly-differentiated cells: 'tumors.' When things go wrong (often in senescence of the organism), with the nuanced overlay that characterizes Metazoa 2.0, the system may revert to the ancient, more robust way of building multicellular assemblages—Metazoa 1.0. The result is cancer. In evading one layer of genetic regulation—turning proto-oncogenes into oncogenes—cancer mutations uncover a deeper, older layer of genes that code for behaviors that are often able to outsmart our best efforts to fight them. The idea of a pre-existing cancer toolkit is not new, but its adoption has been tentative: "Maybe the information for inducing cancer was already in the normal cell genome, waiting to be unmasked" (Weinberg 2007, pg 79). We thus argue that cancer cells are not newly evolved types of cells, but heirs to an ancient toolkit and a basic mode of survival that is deeply embedded in multicellular life. Cancer, like a lazy poet, when called upon to produce new poems, reaches into his trunk of old poems and pulls one out at random, often finding a good poem, popular a billion years ago. These poems are not shoddy, inefficient, preliminary doggerel, but elaborate compositions with pathways that took millions of years to evolve. Some of these pathways are still in active use in healthy organisms today. For example, some of these genes are active during embryogenesis and wound-healing. Others have fallen into disuse, but remain latent in the genome, awaiting reactivation. One might say that the appearance of tumors in the body is a manifestation of the inner Metazoan 1.0 in all of us.

Regarding cancer as the 'default option' for multicellularity is reminiscent of a computer that may start up in Safe Mode if it has suffered either a hardware or a software malfunction. Organisms may suffer mechanical damage such as wounding or inflammation (hardware injury), or genetic damage such as DNA base pair mis-copying (software injury), and as a result, they flip to Safe Mode, unlocking the ancient toolkit of Metazoa 1.0. Just as a computer deals with this crisis by performing system checks and corrections, so too will modern organisms run through a collection of reviews and strategies to repair the damage. If DNA cannot be repaired, there are secondary DNA repair mechanisms. If these fail and the cell begins to proliferate, cell signaling and growth inhibitors try their luck. If these fail to stop proliferation, there is another line of defense—apoptosis (programmed cell death). There is also the immune system. If all of these fail, the outcome is malignant, uncontrolled growth. It is because cancer is the Metazoan 1.0 default option that it is relatively easy to start and hard to stop. Cancer can be triggered in a wide variety of ways, but once it becomes established, it is extremely hard to reverse. That is, cancer can be treated, for example, by destroying tumors, but turning cancer cells back into healthy cells remains a major challenge (Wang et al. 2010). The source of this asymmetry is not hard to find. It took more than a billion years to evolve the eukaryotic genes present in Metazoa 1.0 and approximately another billion years to evolve the sophisticated genetic and epigenetic overlay that led to Metazoa 2.0. It is much easier to inactivate a gene or destroy a complex negative feedback loop than it is to evolve one. This asymmetry makes healthy cells vulnerable to mutations that wreck the delicate machinery of cellular cooperation, thereby reactivating pre-existing ancestral genes. But—and this point should be stressed—such mutations are ineffective, over somatic time scales, at evolving any truly new adaptive features.

Problems with the 'rogue cell' hypothesis. It is sometimes remarked that cancer is a collection of rogue cells, or selfish cells, that recapitulate the world of single cellularity (Merlo et al. 2006). This is superficially plausible. Single-celled eukaryotes obey a simple imperative – replicate, replicate. By contrast, multicellularity demands that individual cells subordinate their selfish agenda to the requirements of the organism as a whole. In modern complex organisms, this hierarchy is accomplished via the aforesaid command and control systems. It is the job of these systems to regulate cell differentiation and proliferation, so as an embryo develops, distinctive tissues and architectures emerge in an organized way and become compartmentalized. The organism functions with a high degree of cooperation between these components. Some organs, such as the stomach, require rapid cell replication to replenish cells sloughed off by wear and tear, while others, such as the brain, have a slow rate of turnover. So long as individual cells replicate according to the organ to which they belong, and both receive and obey the replication commands from the genetic and epigenetic systems, all is well. But it is a hallmark of cancer that malignant cells ignore the normal signals that control replication and apoptosis, and instead, they thrive outside their organ of origin. They may invade the extra-cellular matrix, work their way through vessel walls into the blood or lymphatic systems, become mobile, and then colonize other organs in the body (a process known as metastasis). In short, they behave as a gang of selfish rogue cells. This simplistic account, however, ignores more than a billion years of transitional forms between single-celled eukaryotes and Metazoa 2.0. It ignores Metazoa 1.0. It also fails to hold up to scrutiny. Two problems are immediately apparent. The first is the failure to account for the rather high degree of cooperative organization among cancer cells. The most striking example of this is angiogenesis, in which an entire tumor builds its own blood supply for the common good of all the tumor cells. A more contentious example concerns evidence that a small population of highly malignant cancer cells can be held in check by less malignant cells. Following chemotherapy that targets the dominant population of cancer cells, the restraint is removed, and the more malignant sub-population is unleashed (Eikenberry et al. 2010). Similarly, surgically removing a primary tumor can result in the sudden flourishing of metastatic tumors. Cancer cells are known to exchange chemical signals with each other and with the surrounding tissues, so some degree of cooperation is not unexpected. In this respect, neoplasms resemble ecosystems, consisting of a heterogeneous population of types, rather than a collection of fiercely competitive individuals. To be sure, there is competition, but there is also a certain degree of cooperation and division of labor—exactly what one might expect from Metazoa 1.0.

The second major problem with the rogue cell hypothesis comes when trying to explain cancer's remarkable ability to deploy a formidable array of survival tricks, sometimes all at once. Hallmarks of cancer include the silencing of tumor suppressor genes, switching off apoptosis and anoikis (programmed death when cells detach from the extracellular matrix), switching off senescence by manufacturing enzymes to repair eroding telomeres (Hanahan, Weinberg 2000), evading the immune system by removing surface receptors, dramatically changing the viscoelastic properties of cells to facilitate motility, invasion, and colonization (Butcher et al. 2009). Cancer has also been detected secreting corrosive enzymes to dissolve through organ membranes, thus permitting the cells to enter the blood and lymphatic circulatory systems and spread around the body, thriving in hypoxic conditions by switching off the normal oxidation–phosphorylation metabolism of healthy cells and using the glycolytic cycle instead (the so-called Warburg effect, Warburg 1956), tolerating the resulting low pH conditions far better than healthy cells, shielding themselves from the 'alien cell' alarm signals from organs they invade, manufacturing their own mitogenic signals and growth factors to make them independent of chemical replication signals (Hanahan, Weinberg 2000). Other activities include altering the physical and chemical properties of the extracellular matrix and other host tissues to optimize tumor growth and survival, and accelerating genetic instability to evolve immunity in changing conditions, while rapidly adapting the cytoskeleton dynamics to enable mitosis to operate across a range of karyotypes, including full-blown aneuploidy. The conventional explanation for this multi-faceted armory is straightforward Darwinian evolution, not among species, but inside the host organism, among competing sub-populations of cells within the neoplasm (Merlo et al. 2006). This is called the 'internal' Darwinism hypothesis. In essence, the foregone list of traits is attributed mostly to independent, random mutations and the trial and error of normal Darwinian evolution. The evolution of these survival traits is facilitated by the rapid rate of mutation of cancer cells, combined with strong selective pressure as the organism 'fights back' (or a patient undergoes chemotherapy). As a result, an initially small sub-population of cancer cells that might, by chance, have evolved a trick or two to stymie the next threat (e.g., hypoxia, the immune system, membrane confinement, chemotherapy) are able to exploit their selective advantage and multiply. Then a sub-population of this new population evolves the next trick, and so on, step-by-step, so that, by the time the cancer reaches full malignancy, it possesses a large gamut of survival traits and is virtually indestructible.

Problems with 'internal' Darwinism. The appeal to 'internal' Darwinism to account for the multiplicity of cancer traits as merely 'lucky accidents' of evolution (unlucky for the patient, of course) falls short of a full explanation. It is a fundamental tenet of evolution that random mutations are almost always deleterious, yet cancer seems to 'get lucky' on a suspiciously large number of occasions. Why do the vast majority of mutations in tumor cells not lead to maladaptation and death, as is the case for healthy cells? Especially striking are the large-scale mutations that create jumbled chromosomes and aneuploid cells—well known features of advanced-stage cancer. These cells typically display gross structural changes, such as highly deformed nuclei accompanied by major chromatin reorganization (Zink et al. 2004). Nevertheless, such cells seem not only to survive with their chaotic karyotypes, but also to be remarkably robust (Ao et al. 2008). It appears that, rather than fatally disrupting the elaborate central machinery of cells, these drastic mutations have the opposite effect, of conferring enhanced survivability. "The acquisition of extra copies of one chromosome and the loss of another can create a genetic configuration that somehow benefits the cancer cell" (Weinberg 2007, p 11). This paradox has a ready explanation, however, in light of the atavism hypothesis. The reason that the gross random mutations are far less damaging than one might expect is because the mutations have the effect of short-circuiting the cell's delicate regulatory mechanisms, causing the cell to default to the powerfully adaptive and robust ancient toolkit. Some of the tools are regulatory transcription factors and homeobox genes. Once triggered, they can set in motion the orderly deployment of a succession of survival tricks, including those that propagate colonies of non-differentiated (or very weakly differentiated) cells needed a billion years ago. The reason that newly-reacquired, old ancestral talents are able to benefit cancer cells dwelling within multicellular organisms is that much of the basic biochemistry has remained unchanged over the last billion years of evolution, and the ancestral talents are still useful to cells that do not obediently conform to the organism's newer agenda. Of course, there is a limit to the degree of genetic scrambling that can be tolerated. This model predicts a Goldilocks zone: too few mutations and the cell functions normally, too many and it dies. At some moderate level, normal functional cooperation is lost, but the older genes and a more laissez-faire regulatory regime take over to ensure the cell's survival. It seems very likely that the large majority of severe mutations kill the cells, but there is clearly a selection effect at work; cells that die here and there are cleaned away and are not noticed. Similarly, mild genetic damage that does not seriously compromise the cell's normal functionality, even when widespread across the genome, goes unnoticed, unless discovered through sequencing studies. In between are genetically altered cells with reactivated Metazoan 1.0 genes, and deactivated Metazoan 2.0 cooperation genes. These are cancer cells, and after proliferating to a ~109-cell tumor, they attract attention.

The explanation of cancer as an atavism that short-circuits the Metazoa 2.0 regulatory system and unleashes the suppressed Metazoa 1.0 system receives support from the amazing pleiotropy of some enzymes, and as has been realized recently, some micro-RNAs (miRNAs). Thus the enzyme COX-2 and the miRNA known as miR-31 have been found to control not just one, but a collection of tumorigenic factors. Such remarkable efficiency and economy would be deeply puzzling if it arose from a few decades of internal Darwinism, but it makes perfect sense if it had been honed by evolution over an extended period of time to form an optimized package that constitutes a type of on–off switch for a set of previously adaptive traits.

Another problem with the 'internal' Darwinian account of cancer was pointed out by Bernards and Weinberg (2002a) and concerns the spread of cancer through the body of the host organism. Merlo et al. (2006) summarize the problem: "Metastasis requires that cells leave the primary tumor, but few such cells successfully colonize a distant organ. This leads to a paradox: metastatic clones should have a fitness disadvantage relative to non-metastatic clones in the primary tumor owing to the loss of the progeny that emigrate." Bernards and Weinberg (2002b) offer a tentative explanation based on a 'pre-ordained' correlation between some earlier acquired advantageous genes and the genes that empower metastasis: "... the tendency of a tumor eventually to metastasize is already pre-ordained by the spectrum of mutations that progenitor cells acquire relatively early in tumorigenesis; that is some cancers start out 'on the wrong foot' ... the mutant genes that are known to confer Darwinian selective advantages early on may be the same genes that, further down the line, empower metastasis."

The metastatic paradox is immediately resolved, however, by the atavism hypothesis, because the metastatic phase is internally pre-programmed from the start, and does not emerge via a random 'internal' Darwinian process within the host organism. If the relevant genes are not acquired via random mutations, but are already latent as a package in the genome, ready to be reactivated by a 'spectrum of mutations,' then the 'pre-ordained' nature of metastasis is no longer a mystery. The issue of 'starting out on the wrong foot,' then, simply means that a relatively early genetic or epigenetic mutation opens up access to a pre-existing adaptation for colony formation which manifests itself as the colony-forming abilities of metastatic cancer. The genetic or epigenetic mutations that open up access to pre-existing adaptations can be caused by chronic inflammation, viral infections, or other environmental causes. Because of their pre-existing nature, cancer adaptations should more accurately be called exaptations (Gould, Vrba 1982).

Here, an analogy might be helpful. Cancer's acquisition of ancient traits could be compared to the memory card game in which all the cards are laid out in pre-arranged order face down, and then turned over one by one at random. Initially, the distribution of face-up cards looks chaotic, but once a large subset of the cards is turned over, the order becomes apparent. The emergence of pre-existing order by random uncovering is clearly vastly more efficient than the generation of the same order *ab initio* by a Darwinian process of blind trial and error. Of course, the pre-existing order represented by cancer genes (the toolkit) was the product of a Darwinian process, but one that took place, not in the host organism over a few years, but in its ancestors hundreds of millions of years ago. Thus, we distinguish between acquiring genes from parents (Darwinian evolution, vertical gene transfer), acquiring genes from peers (Lamarckian evolution, horizontal gene transfer), and reactivating the genes of distant ancestors (the atavism known as cancer). There is no claim that internal Darwinism is irrelevant to the progression of neoplasms. Rather, it is asserted that atavistic transformations are a relatively rare part of normal Darwinian evolution, but that they play the dominant role in the progression of cancer.

Phylogenetic tests of the atavism hypothesis. If tumors are a type of living fossil from the era of Metazoa 1.0, it would be expected to find genetic and even fossil evidence. Extant organisms that branched off close to the transition zone between Metazoa 1.0 and Metazoa 2.0 may offer clues. Significantly, the polyp Hydra, the basal eukaryote referred to earlier in connection with the oncogene 'myc,' has the power to regenerate itself, in a cancer-like manner, from a tiny fragment, and can go on doing so seemingly-indefinitely. This ability is reminiscent of the immortalization seen in cancer cells, where the regulated cell divisions of somatic cells undergo an atavistic transformation to their previous less-regulated, pre-multicellular, proto-colonial reproductive regime. Sponges also represent a very ancient form of multicellular life (Brocks, Butterfield 2009), but lack certain features to qualify them for inclusion in the standard definition of eumetazoa (which is being calling Metazoa 2.0 here). The recent sequencing of the Great Barrier Reef demosponge Amphimedon queenslandica (Harcet et al. 2010), supports the hypothesis presented in this paper. It was possible to identify parts of the genome responsible for rudimentary cell cooperation, including cell–to-cell adhesion and, crucially, the regulation of cell proliferation. In effect, the latter are ancient tumor suppressor genes, dating back as far as multicellularity itself. The cancer-as-atavism hypothesis predicts that future phylogenetic studies will find that many oncogenes (the genes that malfunction in the Metazoa 2.0 toolkit) will be found to have evolved during the Metazoa 1.0 to Metazoa 2.0 transition that occurred between 1.3 billion and 600 million years ago. It is apparent that important new insights into the nature of cancer are increasingly coming from efforts, such as this, which seek to correlate the details of the phylogenetic evolution that led to multicellularity, with oncogenes, tumor suppressor genes, and specific mutations that lead to cancer. For example, Srivastava et al. (2010) compared the genomes of organisms that diverged about a billion years ago from the lineage that led to bilaterians and chordates (Srivastava et al. 2008, Putnam et al. 2007, 2008). By looking at the differences in the genomes of representative species at increasing depths in our phylogenetic tree, eumetazoa, metazoa, holozoa, opisthokonta, and multicellular eukaryotes, Srivastava et al. and Putnam et al. were able to establish a preliminary chronology for the order in which the genes associated with multicellularity evolved. These are the genes for cell cycling, growth signaling, apoptosis, and cell differentiation—genes that, when malfunctioning, are implicated in cancer. Recent work by Domazet-Lozo and Tautz (2010) on the phylostratigraphic tracking of cancer genes also lends supports to our cancer-as-atavism hypothesis in that their work establishes a closer link between cancer and the emergence of multicellularity. By identifying and mapping the chronology of the evolution of cell differentiation and cooperation, it may simplify the understanding of the currently forbiddingly complex toolkit of cancer. Since each organism possesses pathways toward cellular differentiation that are initially identical and then branch off (Sulston, Horvitz 1977), it is possible to postulate that the progression of cancer in each cell type will be correlated with the reverse order in which they differentiated. That is, the order in which the effects of mutations can be observed in cells during the progression of cancer should reflect reverse phylogenetic history, in loose analogy with Haekel's maxim that 'ontogeny recapitulates phylogeny.' Ontogeny recapitulates phylogeny largely because mutations inserted later in a developmental pathway do less harm than those inserted earlier (Gould 1977). When genes are eliminated, the consequences vary. Ancient genes are more likely to play a fundamental role than more recently evolved genes, so the consequences of disabling the former tend to be more drastic and likely to lead to cell death.

The prediction can be tested by genomic studies of cancer progression to discover any preferential ordering of traits; for example, is the switching off of apoptosis before or after the secretion of membrane-dissolving proteins or the activation of metastatic pathways? And if there is a preferential sequence, does it reflect the phylogenetic order of the evolution of the genes responsible for these transitions (Mann 2010)? Of course, the postulated correlation may be hidden amid noise, given the high degree of genetic instability in cancer cells, but may nevertheless be discernible in a broad systematic analysis.

One way to embark on such an analysis is to study the development of cancer in representative organisms with different numbers of cell types that branched off from human lineage at increasing depths. Vertebrate blastulas, for example, differentiate into 225 cell types. Invertebrate laterian blastula (e.g., Drosophila, Caenorhabditis elegans) differentiate into 50–100 cell types, while Nematostella and Amphimedon have 10–15 cell types. The placozoan Trichoplax has only 5 cell types (Srivastav et al. 2010). The complexity of cancer in a species should reflect the number of cell types in that species. It would be expected, for example, that Trichoplax, Nematostella, or Amphimedon might suffer in old age from much simpler cancers, the simplicity of which might make them easier to study and control. If large numbers of individuals can be found with cancer within these earlier diverged clades, then it may be possible to study the genomic progression of simpler cancers, based on the malfunctioning of fewer, more basal oncogenes. Plants and fungi are also multicellular eukaryotes, and have also evolved intercellular cooperation mechanisms. There should be an analog of cancer for plants and fungi, but not a great deal is known about this (for example, Sachs 1991). Humans' common ancestor with plants lived 1.6 billion years ago (Hedges, Kumar 2009) and was probably a facultatively colony-forming protist. Some of the earliest genes of cooperation probably evolved around this time and can be identified by the comparative genomics of basal multicellular eukaryotes. This common ancestor with fungi lived 1.3 billion years ago. The deepest-rooted fungi (the chytrids such as Neocallimastigomycota, Blastocladiomycota, and Chytridiomycota) have flagellated motile spores similar to choanoflagellates (basal Holozoans, see King et al. 2008). By comparing the genomes of many species of basal fungi with many species of basal holozoans, and obtaining their branching order in the phylogenetic tree, it should be possible to build a comprehensive account of the evolution of the genes of cellular cooperation between 1.3 and 1.0 billion years ago. This would extend the work of Srivastava et al. (2010) by using more basal metazoan species to obtain a higher time resolution, more statistically robust phylogenetic branching order, and therefore, more robust conclusions about the order of evolution of the genes that enable multicellularity. Extant organisms most similar to these ancestral forms may be found among colonial choanoflagellates, which gate in tumor-like colonies of undifferentiated or weakly-differentiated cells. One might also wonder whether there are fossils dating from the pre-Ediacara era that display the general type of morphology associated with some modern tumors (for example, Maloof et al. 2010). Because tumors are only loosely organized and highly heterogeneous, such a comparison would not be easy, but certain basic features may be discernible. Morphological classification using fractals offers a possible scheme (Baish, Jain

2000). It would also be interesting to discover whether Metazoa 1.0 evolved in hypoxic and low pH conditions—cancer's preferred habitat (Semenza 2007).

Implications for cancer therapy. In this chapter, we have argued that regarding cancer as a collection of rogue individual cells randomly evolving increasingly-refractory survival traits within a few years inside the host organism ('internal' Darwinism) is incomplete and possibly misleading. We postulate that the principal mechanism causing cancer is the accumulation of mutations which destroy the genetic regulation that evolved during the evolution of metazoan multicellularity, thereby reactivating an ancient genetic toolkit of pre-programmed behaviors. In terms of therapeutic response, the distinction between rogue cells and cooperatively organized cells is crucial. Rather than attacking tumors indiscriminately ('the only good cancer cells are dead cancer cells'), understanding their origin, managing them and containing them might be a far smarter strategy. Given cancer's formidable complexity and diversity, how might researchers make progress toward controlling it? If the atavism hypothesis is correct, there are new reasons for optimism. The postulated toolkit of Metazoa 2.0, although admittedly complex, is nevertheless a fixed and finite feature of multicellular life. The number of tools in the kit is not infinite. What one cancer learns cannot be passed on to the next generation of cancers in other patients. Cancer is not going anywhere evolutionarily; it begins again in the next patient (see O'Neil 2010). Although cancer may seem like a perpetually moving target, a given cancer has a strictly limited set of atavistic possibilities open to it. Thus, cancer is a limited and ultimately predictable adversary. This understanding of cancer as a limited atavism should engender optimism among oncologists. The anticipated precision of personalized drug therapies will not be infinite. This view contrasts sharply with the open-ended possibilities for cancer implied by the 'internal Darwinism' model.

If the key to controlling cancer lies with the elucidation of the hypothesized finite number of tools in an inherited toolkit, then advances in technology hold great promise. DNA microarrays, the current super-Moore's law of progress in sequencing technology, and the construction of the Cancer Genome Atlas (http://cancergenome.nih.gov) should soon uncover the limits of the essential genomic varieties of cancer and the limits on their temporal progression. When applied to organisms that branched off from human lineage at different depths, this technology should enable researchers to obtain the evolutionary sequence of the cooperative genes that led to multicellularity—not just in metazoans but possibly in fungi and plants as well. With that new basis of understanding, the way to more effectively combat specific cancers will lie open.

References

Ao P, Galas D, Hood L and Zhu X, 2008, *Cancer as robust intrinsic state of endogenous molecular-cellular network shaped by evolution*, Med. Hypotheses, 70, 678–84.

Baish J W, Jain R K, 2000, *Fractals and cancer,* Cancer Res, 60, 3683.

Bernards R, Weinberg R A, 2002a, *A progression puzzle,* Nature, 418 823.

Bernards R, Weinberg R A, 2002b, *Bernards & Weinberg reply,* Nature, 419 560.

Brocks J J, Butterfield N J, 2009, *Early animals out in the cold,* Nature, 457 672–3.

Butcher D T, Alliston T, Weaver V M, 2009, *A tense situation: forcing tumor progression Nat. Rev.,* Cancer, 9, 108–22.

Chen Y et al., 2000, *Conservation of early odontogenic signaling pathways in Aves,* Proc. Natl Acad. Sci, 97, 10044–9.

Domazet-Lozo T, Tautz D, 2010, *Phylostratigraphic tracking of cancer genes suggests a link to the emergence of multicellularity in metazoan*, BMC Biol, 8, 66.

Eikenberry S E, Nagy J D, Kuang Y, 2010, *The evolutionary impact of androgen levels on prostate cancer in a multi-scale mathematical model,* Biol. Direct, 5 24–52.

Gould S J, 1977, Ontogeny and Phylogeny, Harvard UP, Cambridge, MA.

Gould S J, 1980, *Hen's teeth and horse's toes.* Nat. Hist. Mag, 89, 24–6.

Gould S J, Vrba E S, 1982, *Exaptation—a missing term in the science of form*, Paleobiology, 8, 4–15.

Hall B K, 1984, *Developmental mechanisms underlying the formation of atavisms,* Biol. Rev, 59, 89–122.

Hanahan D, Weinberg R A, 2000, *The hallmarks of cancer.* Cell, 100, 57–70.

Harcet M, Roller M, C´ etkovic´ H, Perina D, Wiens M, Müller WEG, Vlahovicˇek K, 2010 *Demosponge EST sequencing reveals a complex genetic toolkit of the simplest metazoans,* Mol. Biol. Evol, doi:10.1093/molbev/msq174.

Harris M P, Hasso S M, Ferguson M W J, Fallon J F, 2006, *The development of archosaurian first-generation teeth in a chicken mutant*, Curr. Biol, 16, 371–7.

Hartl et al., 2010, *Stem cell-specific activation of an ancestral myc protooncogene with conserved basic functions in the early metazoan Hydra*, Proc. Natl Acad. Sci, 107 4051–6.

Hedges S, Kumar S, 2009, The Timetree of Life, Oxford University Press, Oxford.

King N et al., 2008, *The genome of the choanoflagellate Monosiga brevicollis and the origin of metazoans,* Nature, 451 783.

Le Page M, 2007, *The ancestor within*, New Sci, 193 28.

Maloof A C et al., 2010, *Possible animal-body fossils in Marinoan limestones from South Australia,* Nat. Geosci, 3, 653–9.

Mann A, 2010, *Sponge genome goes deep*, Nature, 466 673.

Merlo L M F, Pepper J W, Reid B J, Maley C C, 2006, *Cancer as an evolutionary and ecological process*, Nat. Rev, Cancer, 6, 924–35.

Nesse R M, Williams G C, 1996, Why We Get Sick: The New Science of Darwinian Medicine, Vintage, New York.

O'Neil I D, 2010, *Tasmanian devil facial tumor disease: insights into reduced tumor surveillance from an unusual malignancy*, Int. J. Cancer, 127, 1637–42.

Putnam N H et al., 2007, *Sea anemone genome reveals ancestral eumetazoan gene repertoire and genomic organization,* Science, 317, 86–94.

Putnam N H et al., 2008, *The amphioxus genome and the evolution for the chordate karyotype*, Nature, 453, 1064–71.

Rothschild B M, Tanke D H, Helbling M II, Martin L D, 2003, *Epidemiologic study of tumors in dinosaurs*, Naturwissenschaften, 90, 495–500.

Sachs T, 1991, Pattern Formation in Plant Tissues, Cambridge University Press, Cambridge, p 38.

Semenza G L, 2007, *Hypoxia and cancer*, Cancer Metastasis Rev, 26, 223–4.

Srivastava M et al., 2008, *The Trichoplax genome and the nature of placozoans*, Nature, 454 955–60.

Sriivastava M et al., 2010, *The Amphimedon queenslandica genome and the evolution of animal complexity,* Nature, 466, 720–7.

Sulston J E, Horvitz H R, 1977, *Post-embryonic cell lineages of the nematode,* Devl Biol, 56 110–56.

Suluanov A et al., 2009, *Hypersensitivity to contact inhibition provides a clue to cancer resistance of naked mole-rat*, Proc. Natl Acad. Sc*i,* USA, 106, 19352–7.

Wang J, Xu L, Wang E, Huang S, 2010, *The potential landscape of genetic circuits imposes the arrow of time in stem cell differentiation*, Biophys. J, 99 29–39.

Warburg O, 1956, *On the origin of cancer cells,* Science, 123, 309–14.

Weinberg R A, 1983, *Oncogenes and the molecular biology of cancer*, J. Cell Biol, 97, 1661–2.

Weinberg R A, 2007, The Biology of Cancer, Garland Science, New York,

Zink D, Fischer A H, Nickerson J A, 2004, *Nuclear structure in cancer cells*, Nat. Rev. Cancer, 4, 677–87.

Chapter III

Stress and Cancer Life

Advances in our understanding of psychoneuroimmunologic relationships have also provided important insights that suggest possible mechanisms that could explain some anecdotal observations (Rosch 1960). Unfortunately, some pop psychologists and self-help zealots have gone overboard by implying that the causes of certain types of cancer are usually stress related. Nothing could be crueler than adding to the stress and guilt of cancer patients than by insinuating that their illness, or their failure to improve with treatment, is due to some deficiency in their character (Rosch 1994) or to imply that their sickness may be their own fault in some way. Many of these claims confirm the questions and concerns I originally conveyed to Selye, and should be kept in mind when evaluating extravagant allegations. A "baker's dozen" of these caveats include:

1. How can we reconcile conflicting animal studies and clinical reports demonstrating that stress can both accelerate and retard malignant growth?
2. What are the mechanisms that might mediate relationships between stress and cancer?
3. Of what does "the immune system" consist and where are its constituents located?
4. What are the best ways to measure immune system functions, with respect to responses to stress and susceptibility to cancer?
5. While certain types of stress appeared to lower immune system measurements thought to reflect resistance to cancer (natural killer cell and T cell mitogenic activity), other stressors have an opposite effect.
6. Stress stimulates some endocrine responses that accelerate the growth of certain tumors, but have inhibitory effects on others.
7. How can we explain the observation that all the interventions we use to treat cancer (radiation, hormones, and chemotherapy), also facilitate the development of malignancy?

The most obvious question is "What Is Stress?" There is still no satisfactory scientific definition of stress, despite decades of attempts to decipher this problem (Solve 1976). 'Stress' is a useless term for pragmatic researchers because it represents different things to different people, is different for each of us, and most importantly, often cannot be measured with any significant degree of accuracy. Stress is used interchangeably to denote physical stressors, such as pain, noise, and opposite extremes of temperature, but also to denote emotional states varying from depression and loneliness to anxiety, anger, and hostility. Do all of these have common characteristics that are relevant to cancer?

Similarly, another obvious question is: "What Is Cancer?" Although the term refers to undisciplined and uncontrollable cellular growth, a basal cell carcinoma of the skin is quite different from adenocarcinoma of the lung, prostate, or breast, brain tumors, lymphomas, leukemias, and other malignancies. These all differ markedly with respect to growth rates, metastatic tendencies, and sensitivity to neuroendocrine or immune system influences, particularly those that might be modulated by stress. There are critical concerns when it comes to determining exactly how long a cancer has been present. If a lump in the breast is found to be malignant, when did the cancer start? A month, six months, or years before clinical detection? Such information would be crucial in establishing any temporal relationship with antecedent stress.

Even if we could confirm stress-induced neuroendocrine system, immune system, or other pathways that induce malignant changes, this is not proof that stress can cause cancer. It is essential to emphasize that association, including the association between stress levels and cancer, never proves causation (Rosch 1983). Although there are well-defined risk factors for certain malignancies, this simply signifies some statistical association, rather than proving a causative, or even contributory role (Rosch 1993). However, although it may never be possible to prove that stress can initiate or modify malignant growth, supportive evidence from different disciplines is impressive and compelling in this regard (Pettingale 1985). Since space limitations preclude documenting all of these, ample supplemental references have been provided to supply additional information on specific topics.

Neurohumoral, Immune, and Subtle Energy Influences

Any attempt to explain how stress could affect malignant growth would have to demonstrate germane effects on systemic activities possessing this potential. There is abundant support with respect to immune, humoral, and central nervous system influences. These three integrative networks are intimately involved in regulating adaptive reactions to stress by surveillance of the status of specific parameters, and responding in an expedient and coordinated fashion (Rosch 1959). The numerous interactions between the central nervous and immune systems and their links to stress can be found in several reviews (Bardos 1983). The hypothalamus plays a crucial role in mediating these interactions as well as endocrine responses (Lippman 1980). Many brain neurotransmitters that can influence malignant growth also participate in the humoral response to stress, including melatonin, serotonin, dopamine, and endorphins.

Some types of cancer are very sensitive to hormonal influences. Estrogens, androgens, progestins, glucocorticoids, insulin-like growth factor, prolactin, and iodothyronines can directly modulate neoplastic growth and influence other hormones that affect cancer cells

(Kakidani, 1982). Some of these actions may be direct, such as estrogen suppression of follicle stimulating hormones, whereas others influence hormonal binding or immune responses (Nagy, 1983). Breast and prostate cancer are notoriously hormone-dependent, and manipulating the hormonal environment is a cornerstone of treatment. Steroidal sex hormones can affect tumor growth factors and other immune system activities, and are sometimes used in the treatment of autoimmune disorders (Brown, 1979). Stress profoundly affects key hypothalamic and pituitary peptides that regulate the activity of target endocrine glands that can modify tumor growth (Lippman, 1978). Glucocorticoids and their congeners dramatically influence the progression of leukemias and lymphomas, and levels produced in response to stress can provide similar clinical benefits. The composer Bela Bartok is often cited as an illustration. While dying in the terminal stages of advanced leukemia, he was approached by Serge Koussevitsky, the Conductor of the Boston Symphony Orchestra, who offered him a commission for a new work. Bartok promptly went into an inexplicable remission, which persisted only until the composition had been completed, after which he promptly succumbed to the disease (Levy, 1987). There are numerous other anecdotes similar to this which support Selye's contention about the benefits of a firm faith and powerful purpose. It is doubtful that these are all mediated by increased glucocorticoid activity, but there are other possible explanations.

Lowered immune defenses clearly predispose to the development of malignancy, and conversely, heightened immune resistance is presumed to provide protection. Consequently, reports attempting to show some relationship between stress and cancer try to support this conclusion by demonstrating suppression or stimulation of the immune system (Bovbjerg, 1993). As noted, stress is a semantic snakepit for scientists, who also have concerns about categorizing different cancers as a collective entity with common characteristics. Similar confusion surrounds the immune system. There is an unfortunate tendency to assume that by giving something a name, we have now somehow defined it, and therefore agree on, or understand, what it means. Although the term is used freely and authoritatively, we have only a sketchy grasp of what the immune system comprises, or where each of its varied components is located. There is no distinct global measurement of immune system function. We can assess levels and ratios of T cells, B cells, helper cells, suppressor cells, natural killer cells, and responses to various blastogenic stimuli. We can measure specific immunoglobulins and antibodies in blood, saliva, urine, and cerebrospinal fluid, thymosin, interferons, interleukins, properdin, and other elements or markers. Humoral immune responses occur in minutes or seconds, whereas those that are cell-mediated may not be evident for days and weeks. The same stressor might cause some immune measures to increase while others are simultaneously suppressed or unaffected. The nature of the stressor, its severity, duration, prior exposure, age, sex, race, nutritional considerations, health status, and hereditary factors may all influence immune responses that have been associated with cancer activity (Cramer, 1981). It is essential to consider such variables when evaluating claims about the effects of stress on "immune system function." Very divergent conclusions could be reached depending upon such modifiers and which particular parameters of immune system function are selected. In addition to the central nervous system, humoral, and immune mechanisms, weak electromagnetic forces may also accelerate or depress malignant growth. Nordenström has postulated that there is an electrical circulatory system in the body. Based on this, he has developed an effective treatment program for lung and breast malignancies using very feeble electrical forces, and these impressive results have now been replicated in other centers. Other investigators have now also confirmed that such energies, in conjunction with conventional therapy, can markedly retard or reverse head and neck cancers and brain tumors previously resistant to treatment. It is not inconceivable that similar subtle forces generated within the body may have comparable consequences that could explain spontaneous regression, as well as a variety of other reported relationships between stress and cancer. The concept that there may be psycho-electro-neuro-immunologic responses has been proposed, and may be useful in exploring this possibility.

Historical support. The belief that stress could cause various diseases or influence their course has always been a popular notion. It can be found in all ancient religions and philosophies, and was emphasized in Ayurvedic principles and practices that have persisted for more than 3500 years. The notion that cancer might in some way be related to emotional stress is as old as the history of recorded medicine. 'Cancer' is derived from *karkinos,* the Greek word for crab, which in Latin became "cancer." This apparently stemmed from the observation that the large veins surrounding a tumor resembled the claws of a crab, as evidenced by Galen's description:

> As a crab is furnished with claws on both sides of the body, so in this disease the veins which extend from the tumor represent with it a figure much like a crab.

Four centuries later, Paul of Aegina suggested:

> Cancer is so called because it adheres with such obstinacy to the part it seizes, that like the crab, it cannot be separated from it without great difficulty

Middle English astronomers unfortunately used the term to describe the constellation between Leo the Lion and Gemini the Twins. Thus, the Tropic of Cancer marks the most northern latitude at which the sun can be seen directly overhead, usually at noon around June 22. Although the use of cancer in astrology has no connection with its medical meaning, some superstitious people still believe that anyone born under this Zodiac sign is more predisposed to die of cancer.

In his treatise on tumors, *De Tumoribus,* Galen observed that melancholy women were particularly prone to cancer of the reproductive organs because they had an excess of black bile (Gr. *melas chole).* This may clarify why the earliest (1601) English definition of cancer explained that:

> Cancer is a swelling or sore coming of melancholy bloud, about which the veins appeare of a blacke or swert colour spread in the manner of a creifish (crayfish) claws.

Galen believed that such humors, vital spirits, imagination, blood, muscle, and nerves were all closely linked with one another, in some hierarchical fashion. Thus, thoughts and feelings were constantly circulating through the body, exerting their effects by direct physical contact with particular parts of our anatomy. This was 2000 years before the development of psycho-neuro-immunology as a discipline.

In 1701, the English physician Gendron emphasized the effect of "disasters of life as occasion much trouble and grief" in the causation of cancer. Eighty years later, Burrows attributed the disease to "the uneasy passions of the mind, with which the patient is strongly affected for a long time. Nunn was impressed with the influence of emotional factors on breast tumors [73] and Stern similarly noted that cancer of the cervix in women was more common in sensitive and frustrated individuals. In the mid-1800's, Walshe's *The Nature and Treatment of Cancer* called attention to

> the influence of mental misery, sudden reverses of fortune and habitual gloomings of the temper on the disposition of carcinomatous matter. If systematic writers can be credited, these constitute the most powerful cause of disease.

Towards the end of the century in a study of more than 250 patients at the London Cancer Hospital, Snow concluded that "the loss of a near relative" was an important factor in the development of cancer of the breast and uterus. Numerous additional citations attest to the firm belief of 18th- and 19th-century physicians that stressful states and emotions predisposed to cancer.

We attach particular importance to these commentaries, because the practice of medicine in the last two centuries was quite different from today. This is particularly important with respect to patient encounters, which were much more personalized. Those physicians had to rely more upon eliciting and appraising the significance of the patient's history, environment, emotional makeup, and lifestyle, in contrast to contemporary diagnostic workups, which emphasize sophisticated laboratory tests and imaging procedures. Their education was much more apt to include a strong background in literature, philosophy, history, and other branches of learning concerned with human thought and relations, rather than the prevailing preoccupation with a basic science curriculum. They undoubtedly spent much more time observing patients, and talking to them about intimate family, social, and work relationships, and other potentially pertinent psychosocial influences. Thus, by virtue of educational enlightenment, cultural orientation, and a more personalized approach, they might well be expected to have had a greater sensitivity to any subtle relationships between stress and cancer, than is possible in the frenetic pace of today's high-tech, and often apathetic, practice environment.

Interest was rekindled in this subject in the 20th century with the advent of psychiatry as a specialty, and its emphasis on individual psycho-dynamics. Evans, a Jungian psychoanalyst, again called attention to the link between loss of a close emotional relationship and cancer. Kissen (1969) first noted that there appeared to be similar personality traits in patients with lung cancer that differentiated them from those with other pulmonary diseases, simply by taking a detailed personal history, and later extended these observations to other malignancies. Schmale (1971) was intrigued with the relationship between antecedent stress and cancer of the cervix. Merely by reviewing a personality questionnaire completed by asymptomatic women with suspicious pap smears, they were able to predict, with almost 75% accuracy, those who would subsequently develop cancer. Malignancy was most likely to surface in women with a "helplessness-prone personality" or overwhelming sense of frustration due to some emotional loss or conflict during the preceding six months, and this has recently been reconfirmed (Greene, 1958). Greene carefully studied the life histories of three sets of identical twins, one of whom had died of leukemia. He noted that each one with the disease had experienced an antecedent emotional upheaval not shared by the survivor. In another 15- year study of patients with lymphoma or leukemia, he found that the disease was more apt to occur following emotional loss or separation, which had engendered sustained feelings of anxiety, anger, sadness, or hopelessness (Thomas, 1974).

Thomas's 40-year prospective health study of medical students was designed to determine whether there were any emotional patterns or stressful antecedents that might predict the development of hypertension in later life. It included a variety of psychological assessment techniques including figure drawing and extensive personal and family interviews. Follow-up revealed that there were personality profiles not only for hypertension, but also suicide, mental illness, coronary heart disease, and cancer. Physicians who subsequently developed tumors often tended to be lonely individuals, who had figuratively "lost their parent," or had difficulties in adequately expressing their emotions. Le Shan, (1956) was impressed with similar characteristics seen in cancer patients, and particularly their possible contributory role (LeShan, 1959). Based on a thorough review of the literature and more than two decades of detailed interviews, he concluded that there were three key types of personality characteristics that tended to precede the onset of malignancy:

1. The loss of an important emotional relationship
2. An inability to express anger or resentment
3. An unusual amount of self-dislike and distress

Feelings of hopelessness and helplessness (Auden, 1919). The first item appears to be of particular importance. Various writers and poets have also emphasized this theme, including Tolstoy, Auden, and Sontag. Even the emotional loss of political defeat has been suggested as contributing to the cancers of Napoleon, Ulysses S. Grant, Robert Taft, Hubert Humphrey, and the Shah of Iran.

Animal research support. Animal studies have also demonstrated links between stress and cancer. Investigators in Pavlov's laboratory reported that dogs subjected to severe and chronic stress had a marked tendency to develop malignancies of the internal organs. Riley (1975) studied a strain of mice carrying the Bittner mammary tumor virus. Under normal circumstances, 70 to 80% of the mice can be expected to develop breast cancer within one year. However, routine conditions in animal laboratories can be quite stressful, even in the absence of painful procedures. There is often unexpected and excessive noise, a confined environment, and frequent jarring movement of the racks holding the cages. Such animals have been shown to have much higher levels of stress-related hormones than others maintained under peaceful and quiet conditions. Exposure to pheromones that signal stressful states might also contribute to this. Riley found that when he protected these mice by placing then in protective housing that completely insulated them from all laboratory commotion and potentially-stressful stimuli, only 7% had evidence of tumors at the end of a year. Conversely, the stress of simply periodically rotating litter mates on a turntable resulted in a 92% incidence of breast cancer (Riley, 1979). The growth of transplanted mammary tumors can also be markedly increased by stressing experimental animals with electric shocks (Visintainer, 1959).

Stress is an unavoidable consequence of life, but is most damaging when it is perceived to be completely beyond control. This is an important issue with respect to relationships with cancer, best illustrated by "yoked testing" experiments. In one such study, two matched groups of rats were housed in separated soundproof chambers and subjected to identical electrical shocks delivered in an erratic fashion with respect to time intervals and duration. When a rat in the first group depressed a small lever, it terminated the shock received by it. In the second group, pressing a similar lever did nothing. A third matched group, living under normal laboratory conditions, received no shocks, serving as controls to reflect normal tumor growth in the absence of this stressful stimulus. All of the animals were injected with a dosage of Walker sarcoma virus calculated to induce malignancies in 50% of recipients to determine whether the physical stress of the shock could influence tumor growth. Three out of four rats in the second group, who received shocks over which they had no control, developed malignant tumors. As expected, the incidence of tumors was 50% in the non-shocked group of rats. However, in the first group of rats, who had received identical shocks as the second but were able to exert some control over them, tumors could be found in only one third. The rats in this group had less than half as many tumors as litter mates subjected to the same stress over which they had no control, and one third less than those who had received no shocks at all.

A "fighting attitude" can retard the development of experimental leukemia in mice, and transplanted mammary tumors in female mice, who spontaneously developed an antagonistic or fighting behavior, were also smaller and slower growing than those in more submissive litter mates. A similar phenomenon has been observed in "feisty" females with breast cancer. This may have therapeutic implications, and again suggests that the feeling of being in control can inhibit malignant growth. Other significant effects of stress on the development and growth of cancer in experimental animals have been summarized elsewhere. However, not all researchers agree. Some supportive animal and clinical studies have been criticized because of their design, failure to control for pertinent variables, and contrary findings with respect to results, or presumed mechanisms of action.

Personality and psychosocial stress as precursors to cancer. In addition to the historical citations noted, more recent reports are also replete with references linking stress and cancer. Depression is most frequently cited, and is supported by evidence of concomitant reduction of natural killer cells and other immune system activities (Linn, 1982). Feelings of helplessness, hopelessness, and suppression of emotions, particularly anger, may predispose someone to cancer (Pettingale, 1997). Suppression of anger is associated with higher serum immune globulin-A levels, which have been shown to correlate with metastases and mortality rates in breast cancer (Traue, 1993). Stress can also affect the metastatic spread of other tumors (Derogatis, 1979).

Increased antecedent stress as assessed by the magnitude of life change events has been reported to be associated with a greater subsequent incidence of certain cancers (Stephenson, 1954). The most stressful life change event is the death (loss) of a spouse, and significantly higher mortality rates for cancer and other leading causes of death have been reported in bereaved survivors over the following 6 to 12 months after the death of a spouse (Schneider, 1984). Several studies have demonstrated concurrent impaired immune function, especially depression of T cell mitogenic and natural killer cell activity during this time period

(Pettingale, 1989). The next three most stressful life change events – divorce, marital separation, and death of a close family member – also reflect emotional losses, and are similarly associated with higher cancer mortality rates. Decreased immune defenses may accompany such losses, and can even be seen in workers who lose their jobs and remain unemployed. Psychosocial stresses such as poverty, social isolation, and low societal status, appear to be risk markers for malignancy. Conversely, the incidence of cancer appears to be unusually low in schizophrenic and certain other psychiatric patients, possibly because they do not consider such situations as stressful, or they may be unable to experience the normal feelings and emotions associated with loss and separation.

Various constellations of personality traits seem to be connected with increased cancer tendencies, and possibly predispose persons to behaviors and lifestyles that are risk factors, or render individuals more susceptible to the effects of stressful life change events. So called "Type C" cancer-prone patients have been characterized as cooperative, conforming, compliant, and unassertive, with a tendency to suppress negative emotions, particularly anger. This characteristic of "pathological niceness" is commonly encountered in cases of malignant melanoma, which is also often associated with increased antecedent stress.

African antelopes and the teleology of evolution. The loss of important emotional relationships clearly constitutes the most stressful life change events. As emphasized above, they also represent the most common emotional and psychological precursors of cancer. Could there be some causal relationship between psychological loss and cancer? Implicit in Cannon's "fight or flight" theory is the teleological premise that our automatic and uncontrollable responses to stress have been steadily sharpened over the lengthy course of evolution. It is posited that they represent adaptive changes that were essential for the survival of our antediluvian ancestors who faced life-threatening physical challenges. The outpouring of adrenalin and stimulation of the sympathetic nervous system resulted in pupillary dilatation to promote better vision, quickened clotting to reduce blood loss from lacerations or internal hemorrhage, a rise in blood pressure and heart rate to increase blood flow to the brain and facilitate decision making, increased blood sugar and lipid levels from the breakdown of carbohydrate and fat stores to furnish more fuel for energy, and numerous other responses that were purposeful for primitive man. The shunting of blood flow away from the gut, where it was not immediately needed for digestive purposes, to the large muscles of the arms and legs provided greater strength for fight in combat, or flight from a scene of potential peril. However, the nature of stress for modern man is not some physical encounter with a saber toothed tiger or warring tribe every few months but rather an array of psychological and emotional threats and challenges which may occur several times daily. The tragedy is that these stressors trigger automatic, archaic, "fight or flight" responses, which are no longer purposeful or appropriate. Repeatedly invoked, it is not difficult to understand how they could contribute to such "Diseases of Civilization" as hypertension, diabetes, heart attacks, strokes, peptic ulcers, muscle spasms, etc. Many of our responses to stress seem senseless, and it may be difficult to appreciate how they could ever have been beneficial. When severely frightened, some people feel their "flesh crawl," develop "goose bumps," or the hairs on the back of the neck "stand up." Although all of these are useless for us, the "flying fur" on the arched back of an aroused cat makes it appear more ferocious to an assailant. Similarly, the stimulation of those same arrector pili muscles is responsible for the "bristling quills" of the porcupine, which is a very effective defense mechanism. Thus, all of our instantaneous, instinctive, reflexive responses to stress undoubtedly served some useful purpose during the lengthy course of human evolution. It is equally apparent that we may often overreact to a stressful stimulus with healing consequences that prove harmful. We see this in the occasional development of disfiguring keloids due to excessive scar formation, and when lip cancer develops in clay pipe smokers, in an attempt to repair heat-damaged tissue.

There are other instances where adaptational evolutionary responses may ultimately prove pernicious. In a review article on Selye's concepts of "Stress" and "Diseases of Adaptation" over 33 years ago, we referred to the theory of "opportunism" in the evolutionary process. This refers to the organism's response to fill a need with whatever means are available, even if the long-term consequences prove undesirable. The illustration cited at that time was the tremendous variation in the development of distinctive horns by some 23 species of African antelopes. The horns of the kudu are prohibitively unwieldy, while those of the duiker are obviously too small to be effective. As one examines the different deviations that have evolved in others, their divergent anatomical configurations and functional capabilities do not appear to serve any rational adaptive purpose. If I were to rewrite that article today, I would choose the development of malignancy in man as perhaps a more dramatic example of "opportunism" in the evolutionary process, for the following reasons.

As one descends the phylogenetic scale, the incidence of malignancy decreases progressively. Cancer does not occur in primitive forms of life. Conversely, the ability of the organism to regenerate injured or lost tissues increases proportionately. Simple organisms, including some invertebrates, have the ability to sever parts of their anatomy when they are injured. This capability would have survival value only if the animal possessed an equally remarkable ability to regenerate the cast off portion from available cell remnants. A starfish can restore a lost appendage, and the newt will grow a new tail or leg if it is severed, or can even cause its mechanical release to escape a predator. This restorative capability is not retained in humans, although the spleen does possess unusual regenerative potential.

It is believed that some malignant responses in man may represent an atavistic, vestigial remnant of this primordial, purposeful, regenerative trait. When we suffer a loss or injury, attempts at replacement could well be activated, as they are in lower life forms. Unfortunately, this new growth (neoplasia) may prove to be harmful rather than helpful. Experiments with chemicals that cause cancer when applied to the human skin or injected into rodents support this hypothesis. When these same carcinogens are injected into the leg of a newt, a new accessory limb starts to grow at that site, rather than a tumor. If injected into the epithelial iris tissue of the eye, the newt will regenerate a new lens. Thus, the identical carcinogenic stimulus can produce either purposeful regeneration or a malignant growth, depending upon the evolutionary development of the organism.

It is interesting that the sole exception to this in humans is the spleen. Years after its surgical removal, remnants of functioning splenic tissue are often found, a phenomenon that has been referred to as the "born again spleen." The spleen is also the only organ in humans that does not give rise to spontaneous cancer, suggesting that its response to loss has been preserved as purposeful regeneration. Small accessory spleens, or spleniculi, are not uncommon, and in rare cases, several hundred may be present in or around the gastrointestinal tract. This represents a reversion to a more primitive condition, in which splenic tissue is not located in a single organ, but instead is scattered throughout the gut. Thus, from the standpoint of embryology and comparative anatomy, the spleen retains certain ancient attributes that may explain its unique freedom from cancer, as well as its remarkable regenerative capacity.

The leap from physical to emotional loss should not be too troublesome. The ability to regenerate lost or injured tissue in lower forms of life obviously involves something more than a simple local response. The message that tissue has been lost, irritated, or damaged must be relayed to higher centers in the central nervous system. These could initiate coordinated restorative activities, most likely involving the integration of central nervous system, humoral, and immune system mechanisms. With man's highly developed cerebral cortex, emotional loss may well be perceived as being an equally significant or even greater stress than physical privation. The same reparative signals may be activated, but our responses are anomalous and aberrant. Our strivings to stimulate purposeful replacement are futile and fruitless, and any resultant new growth is apt to be in the form of malignant neoplasia.

Selye was unusually enthusiastic about this theory, and emphasized it and associated concepts in his Foreword to *Cancer, Stress and Death:*

> Perhaps, as Paul Rosch of New York has suggested, cancer might even be an attempt by the human organism to regenerate tissues and organs and even limbs, as lower animals are able to do spontaneously. Going further, one might say that "the ultimate health of the organism, like that of society, appears to depend on how well or appropriately its constituent units communicate with one another

Cancer and civilization. In keeping with Selye's assignment, the title of my paper was "Stress and Cancer: A Disease of Adaptation?" In retrospect, "A Disease of Civilization" might have been a more appropriate subtitle. This may suggest some allusion to smoking, air pollution, the proliferation of putative cancer-causing substances such as asbestos, depletion of the ozone layer, radiation hazards, or other current carcinogenic concerns. However, what I wish to refer to are psychosocial stresses that were evident long before these 20th-century problems. This concept is not new, and was proposed over 150 years ago in Tanchou's 1843 *"Memoir on the Frequency of Cancer"* delivered to the French Academy of Sciences:

> M. Tanchou is of the opinion that cancer, like insanity, increases in a direct ratio to the civilization of the country and of the people. And it is certainly a remarkable circumstance, doubtless in no small degree flattering to the vanity of the French *savant,* that the average mortality rate from cancer in Paris during 11 years is about 0.80 per 1000 living annually, while it is only 0.20 in London! Estimating the intensity of civilization by these data, it clearly follows that Paris is four times more civilized than London.

Bainbridge's *The Cancer Problem,* noted:

> Man in his primeval condition has been thought to be very little subject to new growth, particularly to those of a malignant character. With changed environment, it is claimed by some, there came an increase in susceptibility to cancerous disease, this susceptibility becoming more marked as civilization develops.

Hoffmann's treatise *The Mortality of Cancer Throughout the World,* a global survey conducted under the auspices of the Prudential Life Insurance Company, emphasized:

> The rarity of cancer among native races (primitive races) suggests that the disease is primarily induced by the conditions and methods of living which typify our modern civilization ... A large number of medical missionaries and other trained medical observers, living for years among native races throughout the world, would long ago have provided a more substantial basis of fact regarding the frequency of occurrence of malignant disease among the so-called uncivilized races, if cancer were met with among them to anything like the degree common to practically all civilized countries. Quite the contrary, the negative evidence is convincing that, in the opinion of qualified medical observers, cancer is exceptionally rare among the primitive peoples including the North American Indians and the Eskimo population of Labrador and Alaska

This was substantiated by the African medical missionary, Dr. Albert Schweizer:

> On my arrival in Gabon in 1913, I was astonished to encounter no cases of cancer. I cannot, of course, say positively that there was no cancer at all; but like other frontier doctors, I can only say that if any cases existed, they must have been quite rare. In the course of the years, we have seen cases of cancer in growing numbers in our region. My observations incline me to attribute this to the fact that the natives are living more and more after the manner of the whites.

Similarly, the celebrated anthropologist and Arctic explorer, Vilhjalmur Stefansson, in his book which actually was titled *Cancer: Disease of Civilization?,* noted the absence of cancer in the Eskimos upon his arrival in the Arctic, but a subsequent increase in the incidence of the disease as closer contact with white civilization was established. He quoted Sir Robert McCarrison, a physician who had studied 11,000 Hunza natives in Kashmir from 1904 to 1911. They not only enjoyed unusual longevity, but preserved their youthful physique and appearance well into their sixties and seventies. McCarrison attributed the absence of cancer to the fact that they were "endowed with a nervous system of notable stability" (resistant to stress), and "far removed from the refinement of civilization."

Hay's *Cancer: A Disease of Either Election or Ignorance,* commented:

> A study of the distribution of cancer, among the races of the entire earth, shows a cancer ratio in about proportion to which civilization living predominates; so evidently something inherent in the habits of civilization is responsible for the difference of cancer incidence compared with the uncivilized races and tribes. Climate has nothing to do with this difference, as witness the fact that tribes living naturally will show a complete absence until mixture with more civilization, even so does cancer begin to show its head.

In *Malignancy and Evolution,* Roberts wrote, "I take the view commonly held that, whatever its origin, cancer is very largely a disease of civilization." He was referring to opinions such as those expressed in Moore's *The Antecedents of Cancer,* that "connect the progress of civilization with the increase of cancer which has remained an incontestable theory to the present day"; Banks' contention that "cancer is on the increase in this country. Is it possible that this is coincident with our full habit of living as a people?"; Powell's *The*

Pathology of Cancer: "There can be little doubt that the various influences grouped under the title of civilization play a part in producing a tendency to Cancer"; and Hooker's *Eclecticism in Cancer Therapy,* which urged less emphasis upon research in artificially induced cancer in laboratory animals, and more emphasis upon the observation of people:

> There is, as a matter of fact, a growing group of independent thinkers both lay and professional, who are anything but impressed with the story of the discovery and isolation of the "cancer germ". Mr. Ellis Barker has also written reiterating his views, in common with those of Sir William Arbuthnot Lane, my own and many others, that cancer is a disease of civilization.

One of the most persuasive arguments is to be found in Berglas' *Cancer: Its Nature, Cause and Cure.* Throughout this book runs the theme that cancer is a disease from which primitive peoples are relatively or wholly free, and that we are

> threatened with death from cancer because of our inability to adapt to present day living conditions ... Over the years, cancer research has become the domain of specialists in various fields. Despite the outstanding contributions of scientists, we have been getting farther away from our goal, the curing of cancer. This specialized work, and the knowledge gained through the study of individual processes, has had the peculiar result of becoming an obstacle to the whole. More than thirty years in the field of cancer research have convinced me that it is not to our advantage to continue along this road of detailed analysis. I have come to the conclusion that cancer may perhaps be just another intelligible natural process whose cause is to be found in our environment and mode of life.

In addition to cancer, simple and stable societies are relatively resistant to diabetes, hypertension, peptic ulcer, and other "Diseases of Civilization." However, as Donnison reported in *Civilization and Disease,* this resistance is rapidly lost when established norms and traditions are swept aside by the pressures of civilization. Since the advent of Cro-Magnon, societal groups have progressively increased in size, and changed dramatically with respect to interpersonal relationships and values. Appropriate adaptive alterations have not kept pace with these evolutionary advances with respect to the acquisition of psychological and emotional assets that could facilitate acclimatization to swiftly shifting sociocultural environments. "Social disruption" may also increase susceptibility to tuberculosis and other infectious diseases. [207] It is the rapidity of change which particularly predisposes individuals to inappropriate and damaging coping responses that eventually result in reduced resistance to both physical and emotional disorders. Recent government statistics show a puzzling increase in the incidence of breast cancer in middle-aged females, which may also be related to certain new stresses of "civilization." It has been well established that the younger a woman is when she has her first child or even becomes pregnant, the less likely she is to develop breast cancer. Pregnancy lowers prolactin which stimulates breast tissue growth and promotes breast cancer in experimental animals. As more and more women enter the workforce, they tend to remain single, marry later in life, and decide not to have children or do so only when they are much older. Similarly, the incidence of deadly ovarian cancer is 14 times higher in career-oriented, single working women, compared to a matched group of homemakers. Job stress itself may be a factor, as many women workers have to juggle job responsibilities with being a wife, supermom, single parent, or providing custodial duties for an aged relative. Superimposed on this, there may be sexual harassment, lower compensation than male counterparts despite superior ability and experience, and a dead end when they try to reach the upper rungs of the corporate ladder.

Other demographic groups, including children, adolescents and the elderly are subjected to unique stresses not experienced generations ago, as a consequence of changes imposed by the pressures of contemporary civilization. Key among these are the rapid sociocultural changes that have eroded close family and religious ties, and the sense of belonging, so deftly described by Wolf in his studies of Roseto. These also represent loss of meaningful emotional relationships that may not be fully appreciated, because they are not sudden and dramatic detachments. For today's younger generations, social ties are more often apt to lie in rooting for the same sports team, or being a fan of some rock group, or celebrity, rather than religion, family, or humane and redeeming relationships which are oriented towards, and have the capacity to relieve, loss and suffering.

Bio-psycho-socio-ecological communication, control, and subtle energies. Similarly, civilization also seems to have been responsible for a progressive loss of communication with the cosmos, or nature. Life on earth consists of a hierarchy of living systems that range upward from atoms, molecules, cells, and organs, to people, families, corporations, and societies. Poorly understood communication channels continually connect all these components, as meaningful messages are sent up and down the line. Homeostasis and health are entirely dependent on good communication – good communication not only within the constituency of the internal environment of each system, but also with the external environment at higher and lower levels. These dynamic interrelationships are essential for the preservation of balance, harmony, and homeostasis in the universe. Such a bio-psycho-socio-ecologic perspective must be appreciated to comprehend the complex connections between psychosocial stress and cancer.

As Yamasaki has elegantly demonstrated, the basic problem with the cancer cell is that it no longer communicates properly:

> Cancer can be regarded as a rebellion in an orderly society of cells when they neglect their neighbors and grow autonomously over surrounding normal cells. Since intercellular communication plays an important role in maintaining an orderly society, it must be disturbed in the process of carcinogenesis. Evidence suggests that blockage of intercellular communication is important in the promotion process of carcinogenesis

Selye had previously described this need for cooperative communication in more humanistic terms:

> The indispensability of this disciplined, orderly mutual cooperation is best illustrated by its opposite— the development of a cancer, whose most characteristic feature is that it cares only for itself.

But how does communication take place in the body? The nervous system communicates by direct contact, as adrenergic or cholinergic molecules are released at nerve endings and synapses. Endocrine secretions and neurotransmitter secretions are carried via the bloodstream to selected receptor sites on cell walls at distant locations. Much less is known about the immune system, although it is clear that its conversations include both humoral and hard wired connections. However, in the final analysis, all of these messages are transmitted by means of weak energy transfers across cell membranes. These occur at an atomic rather than a molecular level. It has also become increasingly apparent that the cell membrane is more than a protective shield studded with receptor sites for antibodies, small neuropeptides, and other molecules. It appears to be a powerful signal amplifier that provides an interactive window through which the cell senses and responds to its environment. Some substances can pass freely back and forth through certain channels, but for others, the cell membrane is an impenetrable barrier. When designated molecules fit into special receptor sites, a subtle signal produces a sudden change in electrical tension between the interior and exterior of the cell, allowing a new channel to open for a few thousandths of a second. During this period, although millions of ions pass back and forth, the total current generated is only a few billionths of an ampere! As previously proposed, we believe that cell membranes may have receptor sites for subtle energy signals which react exactly as they would to chemical/molecular stimuli. Electrical stimulation of highly specific areas in the pain pathway produces analgesia, and microinjections of morphine at these precise sites have the identical effect. Injection or stimulation from a few millimeters away is worthless. However, combining suboptimal doses of morphine or electrical stimulation, which alone are too weak to reduce pain, results in a synergistic effect that does provide analgesia. This suggests that for some receptors, the effects of weak electrical stimulation are completely congruent with those of morphine. Furthermore, the specific locations at which either molecular or electrical signals relieve pain are precisely the sites of action of the endorphins. If feeble electrical forces can produce such profound physiologic effects, this might account for the association of malignancy with proximity to high power lines, increased birth defects when electric blankets are used during pregnancy, and a variety of psycho-physiologic effects due to geomagnetic influences, including cancer. Such observations cannot be explained in terms of Newtonian physics, or any form of chemical/molecular communication. It is quite likely that energies of similar magnitude can be generated in the body, which could also affect cell growth and malignant change. *Electroencephalogram (EEG) waves may reflect more than the noise of the machinery of the brain, and possibly represent signals being sent to other parts of the body. Since it is possible to move a cursor on a computer screen solely by deep concentration, it does not seem unreasonable to postulate that mental activities could also affect activities in the body that are sensitive to rent chemical/molecular concept of communication, to a physical/atomic model. Such a paradigm might explain not only regression or spontaneous remission of cancer in patients with a strong determination, but also the placebo effect, faith healing, "therapeutic touch," psychokinesis, telepathy, and other widely acknowledged, but poorly understood, phenomena.*

Pribram (1993) and Bohm (1980) propose that the universe consists of swirls of energy fields that operate in dimensions far beyond our conventional senses. They view the brain as a holographic instrument which mathematically constructs concrete realities by interpreting these energies from another dimension that transcends our current comprehension of time and space. A similar concept was expressed by William Wordsworth in his *Ode On The*

Intimations Of Immortality From Recollections Of Early Childhood, and in recent years, Sheldrake (1992) has provided some scientific support for such beliefs (Kobasa, 1982). The Chinese conceptualization of *"chi"* energy and its role in health and disease has persisted for thousands of years, and is increasingly attracting scientific interest and support. However, *chi* is not only an energy system that flows through acupuncture meridians in the body, but is found in trees, rocks, and all of nature. Hence, the need to add an ecological component to our current bio-psycho-social model of health.

Although we cannot perfectly define stress, all of our research confirms that the sense of being out of control is always distressful. That also happens to be an accurate definition of the cancer cell. It is a cell that is out of control, because it does not communicate properly with its neighbors, or the rest of the organism. A domineering and dogmatic determination, firm and forceful faith, and aggressive attitude all reflect the development of a strong sense of control. These are common themes in reports of patients who triumphed over seemingly fatal malignancies (Kune, 1993). Can this message of control be communicated to cancer cells through unsuspected energy pathways to alter their undisciplined activities? Is it possible to listen in on this conversation? If we understood its vocabulary, could we learn how to emulate, simulate, or stimulate such subtle signals, and to utilize our innate and awesome potential for self-healing?

How can one explain the numerous well-documented cases of spontaneous remission of cancer? Careful studies of such patients suggest that a firm faith and a strong positive belief system is the lowest common denominator (Cole, 1974). Anecdotal, but irrefutable, reports of cancer cures from shrines, faith healers, laetrile®, coffee enemas, acupuncture, macrobiotic diets, and other alternative treatments are difficult to explain. There are numerous reports of cancer regression through the use of various stress reduction or mind-altering techniques, including intense meditation, visual imagery, and hypnosis (Hedge, 1960). Yet, like spontaneous remission, all these cures are extremely rare, and benefits are entirely unpredictable in any given patient. Here again, having a strong faith in anything which the individual believes, and which provides a sense of control, might offer the best explanation. But how are the salutary rewards of faith healing, "therapeutic touch," and the placebo effect mediated? Is there such a thing as psychic healing? How can one explain the well-documented benefits associated with the development of strong social support in patients with cancer and other problems?[1] Conversely, what are the mechanisms involved in the numerous reports of reactivation of dormant cancer following an extremely stressful event, particularly sudden loss? No consistent immune, neuroendocrine, or central nervous system changes have been demonstrated in connection with such effects (Rosch, 1981). Could the answer lie in some latent energy force? Is it possible to learn how to harness this?

The Endemiology of Cancer

We are exposed daily to a host of potential physical carcinogens in the air we breathe or the foods we eat. However, not all smokers develop lung cancer, which also occurs in nonsmokers without any family history of malignancy or other conceivable contributory factor. I would suggest that there may be equally powerful psychosocial carcinogens that exist both in our external and internal milieus. Our current focus is on the epidemiology of cancer, the roots of which connote some external stressor to which the individual has been subjected. What we must now also acknowledge is what might be referred to as the endemiology of cancer, and those factors that influence health which are generated in our internal environment (Rosch, 1986).

Good health is entirely dependent on maintaining the constancy or stability of the internal environment during stress. Walter Cannon coined the term "homeostasis," from the Greek *homios* (similar) and *stasis* (position), to refer to this "steady state" (Canon, 1932). However, the concept of the importance of the internal environment, and the term itself *(milieu interieur)*, originated a half century earlier with the celebrated French physiologist Claude Bernard (1945), often called "The Father of Physiology." Louis Pasteur was a powerful proponent of external causes of disease because of his discovery of pathogenic bacteria. He engaged in many debates about this with Claude Bernard at the prestigious *Academie Française,* where they sat next to one another. However, on his deathbed, Pasteur allegedly stated *"Bernard avail raison. Le germe n'est rien, c'est le terrain qui est tout."* [Bernard was right. The microbe is nothing, the soil is everything] (Pasteur, 1956).

Sir William Osier reported the spontaneous shrinkage of metastases from breast cancer in two women in 1901 (Osier, 1976). It is interesting that the term "spontaneous" is so often used to describe this phenomenon, rather than "unexplained." Spontaneous refers to occurrences that happen without apparent external cause, and are therefore self-generated, as in "spontaneous combustion." Osier often commented that it was more important to know what went on in a patient's head than in his chest, to determine the clinical course of tuberculosis. He also paraphrased Parry's perception that "It is much more important to know what sort of a patient has a disease, than what sort of a disease the patient has (Osier, 1905). This observation, as well as the important role of stress, is being increasingly confirmed in patients with hypertension, coronary heart disease, peptic ulcer, allergic conditions, psoriasis, low back pain, and a variety of mental and emotional disorders. As suggested in this chapter, it may be appropriate to insert cancer near the top of this list of "Diseases of Civilization."

References

Achterberg, J. and Lawlis, G. F., *Imagery of Cancer,* Institute for Personality and Ability Testing, Champaign, IL, 1978.

Achterberg, J., Matthews, S., and Simonton, O. C., Psychology of the exceptional cancer patient—a description of patients who outlive predicted life expectancies, *Psychother. Theory Res. Practice,* 9, 1-21, 1976.

Adelstein, A. M., Life-style in occupational cancer, *J. Toxic. Environ. Health,* 6, 953-962, 1980.

Ader, R., Felten, D. L., and Cohen, N., Eds., *Psychoneuroimmunology,* Academic Press, San Diego, 1991.

Ananth, J. and Bernstein, M., Cancer less common in psychiatric patients, *Psychosomatics,* 18, 44-46, 1977.

Antonovsky, A., *Health, Stress, and Coping: New Perspectives on Mental and Physical Weil-Being,* Jossey-Bass, San Francisco, 1979. Wolf, S., Herrenkohl, R. C., Lasker, J., Egloff, J., Philips, B. U., and Bruhn, J. G., Roseto, Pennsylvania, 25 years later—highlights of a medical and sociological survey, *Trans. Am. Clin. Ciimatoi. Soc.,* 100, 57-67, 1988.

Auden, W. H., *Collected Poems,* Random House, New York, 1991.

Azavedo, E., Svane, G., and Nórdenstrom, B., Radiological evidence of response to electrochemical treatment of breast cancer, *Clin. Radiol.,* 43, 84-87, 1991.

Bagenal, F. S., Easton, D. F., Harris, E., Chilvers, C. E. D., and McElwain, T. J., Survival of patients with breast cancer attending Bristol cancer help centre, *Lancet,* 336, 606-610, 1990.

Bahnson, C. B., Stress and cancer: the state of the art. I, *Psychosomatics,* 21, 975-981, 1980; Stress and cancer: the state of the art. II; *Psychosomatics, 22,* 207-220, 1981.

Bainbridge, W. S., *The Cancer Problem,* Macmillan, New York, 1914. Hoffman, F. L., *Mortality From Cancer Throughout The World,* Prudential Press, Newark, 1916.

Balitsky, K. P., Shmalko, Y. P., and Pinchuk, V G., Stress, cancer: stress modulation of the metastatic process, in *Cancer, Stress, and Death,* 2nd ed., Day, S. B., Ed., Plenum Publishing, New York, 1986, 113-129.

Bammer, K., Stress, spread and cancer, in *Stress and Cancer,* Bammer, K. and Newberry, B. H., Eds., C. J. Hogrefe, Toronto, 1981, 137-163.

Bardos, P., Biziere, K., DeGenne, D., and Renoux, G., Regulation of natural killer activity by the cerebral neocortex, in *Natural Killers: Fundamental Aspects and Role in Cancer,* Serron, B. and Herberman, R. B., Eds., Elsevier, Amsterdam, 1983, 346-359.

Bartrop, R. W., Luckhurst, E., Lazarus, L., Kiloh, L. G., and Penny, R., Depressed lymphocyte function after bereavement, *Lancet,* 1, 834-836, 1977.

Belehradek, J., Orłowski, S., Poddevin, B., Paoletti, C., and Mir, L. M., Electrotherapy of spontaneous mammary tumours in mice, *Eur. J. Cancer,* 27, 73-76, 1991.

Belehradek, M., Domenge, C., Luboinski, B., Orłowski, S., Belehradek, J., and Mir, L. M., Electrotherapy, a new antitumor treatment. First clinical phase l-ll trial, *Cancer,* 72, 3694-3700, 1993.

Ben-Eliyahu, S., Yirmiya, R., Shavit, Y., and Liebeskind, J. C., Stress-induced suppression of natural killer cell cytotoxicity in the rat: a naltrexone-insen- sitive paradigm, *Behav. Neurosci.,* 104, 235-238, 1990.

Berczi, I. and Nagy, E., A possible role of prolactin in adjuvant arthritis, *Arthritis Rheum.,* 25, 591-594, 1982.

Bernard, C., *Introduction to the Study of Experimental Medicine,* Flammarion, Paris, 1945 (Original edition 1865).

Besedovskv, H. O. and Sorkin, E., Network of immune-neuroendocrine interactions, *Clin. Exp. Immunol., 21,* 1-12, 1977.

Besedovskv, H. O. and Sorkin, E., Network of immune-neuroendocrine interactions, in *Hormonal Control of Immune Processes,* James, V. H. T., Ed., Oxford University Press, Amsterdam, 1977, 504-513.

Besedovsky, H. O., Sorkin, E., Felix, D., and Haas, H., Hypothalamic changes during the immune response, *Eur. J. Immunol.,* 7, 323-325, 1977.

Bieliauskas, L. A. and Garron, D. C., Psychological depression and cancer, *Gen. Hosp. Psychiatry,* 4, 187-195, 1982.

Bohm, D., *Wholeness and the Implicate Order,* Routledge and Kegan Paul, London, 1980.

Bolen, J. S., Meditation and psychotherapy in the treatment of cancer, *Psychic,* 4, 19-22, 1973.

Bovbjerg, D. H. and Valdimarsdottir, H., Familial cancer, emotional distress, and low natural cytotoxic activity in healthy women, *Res. Nurse Health,* 16, 395-404, 1993.

Breedis, C., Induction of accessory limbs and of sarcoma in the newt with carcinogenic substances, *Cancer Res.,* 12, 861-866, 1952.

Brown, F., The relationship between cancer and personality, *Ann. NY Acad. Sci.,* 125, 865-875, 1966.

Brown, G., Seggle, J., and Ettigi, P., Stress, hormone responses, and cancer, in *Cancer, Stress, and Death,* Tache, J., Selye, H., and Day, S. B., Eds., Plenum, New York, 1979, 29-39.

Bruhn, J. and Wolf, S., *The Roseto Story: An Anatomy of Health,* University of Oklahoma Press, Norman, 1978.

Bulloch, K., Neuroendocrine-immune circuitry: pathways involved with the induction and persistence of humoral immunity, *Diss. Abstr. Int.,* 41, 4447-B, 1981.

Burrows, J., *A New Practical Essay on Cancer,* London, 1783.

Cannon, W. B., *The Wisdom of the Body,* W. W. Norton, New York, 1932.

Cassell, J., The contribution of the social environment to host resistance, *Am. J. Epidemiol.,* 104, 7-13, 1976.

Cassileth, B. R., Lusk, E. J., Miller, D. S. et al., Psychological correlates of survival in advanced malignant disease?, *N. Engl. J. Med.,* 312, 1551-1555, 1985.

Clawson, T. A. and Swade, R., The hypnotic control of blood flow and pain: the cure of warts and the potential for the use of hypnosis in the treatment of cancer, *Am. J. Clin. Hypn.,* 17, 160-169, 1975.

Cole, W. H., Spontaneous regression of cancer. The metabolic triumph of the host?, *Ann. NY Acad. Sci.,* 230, 111, 1974.

Cooper, C. L. and Faragher, E. B., Psychosocial stress and breast cancer: the inter-relationship between stress events, coping strategies and personality, *Epidemiol. Rev.,* 15, 163-168, 1993.

Cooper, C. L., The social-psychological precursors to cancer, *J. Hum. Stress,* 10, 4-11, 1984.

Cox, T. and Mackay, C., Psychosocial factors and psychophysiological mechanisms in the aetiology and development of cancers, *Soc. Sci. Med.,* 16, 381-396, 1982.

Cramer, D. L., The semantics of cancer, *Int. Med., 2,* 9, 1981.

Cross, R. J., Markesbery, W. R., Brooks, W. H., and Rozman, T. L., Hypothalamic-immune interactions. The acute effect of anterior hypothalamic lesions on the immune response, *Brain Res.,* 196, 79-87, 1980.

Dattore, P. J., Shontz, F. C., and Coyne, L., Premorbid personality differentiation of cancer and non-cancer groups: a test of the hypothesis of cancer proneness, *J. Consult. Clin. Psychol.,* 48, 388-394, 1980.

Derogatis, L. R., Abeloff, M. D., and Melisaratos, N., Psychological coping mechanisms and survival time in metastatic breast cancer, *JAMA,* 242, 1504-1508, 1979.

Derogatis, L. R., Morrow, G. R., Fetting, J., Penman, D., Piasetsky, S., Schmale, A. M., Henrichs, M., and Carnicke, C. L., Jr., The prevalence of psychiatric disorders among cancer patients, *JAMA, 249,* 751-757, 1983.

Donaldson, D. J. and Mason, J. M., Cancer related aspects of regeneration research: a review, *Growth,* 39, 475-496, 1975.

Donnison, C. P., *Civilization and Disease,* William Wood, Baltimore, 1938. Halliday, J. L., *Psychosocial Medicine: A Study of the Sick Society,* W. W. Norton, New York, 1948.

Dubos, R., Biological and social aspects of tuberculosis, *Bull. NY Acad. Med.,* 27, 351, 1951.

Dunbar, F., *Emotions and Bodily Changes,* 4th ed., Columbia University Press, New York, 1954.

Eguchi, E. and Watanabe, K., Elicitation of lens formation from the ventral iris epithelium of the newt by a carcinogen N-methyl-N-nitro-N-ni- trosoguanidine, *J. Embryol. Exp. Morphol.,* 30, 63-71, 1973.

Eli, K., Nishimoto, R., Mediansky, L., Mantel I, J., and Hamovitch, M., Social relations, social support and survival among patients with cancer, *J. Psychosom. Res., 36,* 531-541, 1992.

Evans, E., *A Psychological Study Of Cancer,* Dodd-Mead and Co., New York, 1926.

Eysenck, H. J., Grossarth-Maticek, R., and Everitt, B., Personality, stress, smoking, and genetic predisposition as synergistic risk factors for cancer and coronary heart disease, *Integr. Physiol. Behav. Sci.,* 26, 309-322, 1991.

Eysenck, H. J., Personality, stress, and motivational factors in drinking as determinants of risk for cancer and coronary heart disease, *Psychol. Rep.,* 69, 1027-1043, 1991.

Fauci, A. S., Mechanisms of the immunosuppressive and anti-inflammatory effects of glucocorticoids, *J. Immunopharmacol.,* 1, 1-25, 1978.

Felten, D. L., Cohen, N., Ader, R., Felten, S. E., Carlson, S. L., and Rozman, T, L., Central neural circuits involved in neural-immune interactions, in *Psychoneuroimmunology,* Ader, R., Felten, D. L., and Cohen, N., Eds., Academic Press, San Diego, CA, 1991, 3-18.

Fox, B. H. and Newberry, B. H., *Impact of Psychoendocrine Systems in Cancer and Immunology,* C. J. Hogrefe, Lewiston, NY, 1984.

Fox, B. H., Premorbid psychological factors as related to cancer incidence, *J. Behav. Med.,* 1, 45-133, 1978.

Funch, D. P. and Marshall, J., The role of stress, social support and age in survival from breast cancer, *J. Psychosom. Res., 21,* 177-183, 1983.

Funch, D. P. and Mettlin, C, The role of support in relation to recovery from breast surgery, *Soc. Sci. Med.,* 16, 91-98, 1982.

Gendron, D., Enquiries Into The Nature, Knowledge And Cure Of Cancer, London, 1701.

Gibertini, M., Reintgen, D. S., and Baile, W. F, Psychosocial aspects of melanoma, *Ann. Piast. Surg., 28,* 17-21, 1992.

Gibson, W. T., *The Etiology and Nature of Cancerous and Other Growths,* John Bale Sons & Danielsson, London, 1909.

Gisler, R. and Schenkel-Hulliger, L., Hormonal regulation the immune response. II. Influence of pituitary and adrenal activity on immune responsiveness in vitro, *Cell Immunol., 2,* 646-657, 1971.

Glaser, R., Rice, J., Stout, J. C., Speicher, C. E., and Kiecolt-G laser, J. K., Stress depresses interferon production by leukocytes concomitant with a decrease in natural killer cell activity, *J. Behav. Neurosci,* 100, 675-678, 1986.

Good, R., A., personal communication.

Gordon-Taylor, G., The incomputable factors in cancer prognosis, *Br. Med. J.,* 1, 455, 1959.

Gossarth-Maticek, R., Bastiaans, J., and Kanazin, D. T., Psychosocial factors as strong predictors of mortality from cancer, ischemic heart disease and stroke: the Yugoslav prospective study, *J. Psychosom. Res.,* 29, 167-176, 1985.

Greene, W. A. and Miller, G., Psychological factors and reticuloendothelial disease, *Psychosom. Med., 20,* 124-144, 1958.

Greene, W. A., The psychosocial setting of the development of leukemia and lymphoma, Ann. *NY Acad. Sci.,* 125, 794-801, 1966

Greer, S. and Morris, T., Psychological attributes of women who develop breast cancer: a controlled study, *J. Psychosom. Res.,* 19, 147, 1975.

Greer, S. and Morris, T., The study of psychological factors in breast cancer: problems of method, Soc. *Sci. Med.,* 12, 129-134, 1978.

Greer, S. and Watson, M., Towards a psychobiological model of cancer: psychological considerations, *Soc. Sci. Med., 20,* 773-777, 1985.

Greer, S., Moorey, S., Baruch, J. D. R., Watson, M. et al., Adjuvant psychological therapy for patients with cancer: a prospective randomized trial, *Br. Med. J.,* 304, 675-680, 1992.

Greer, S., Morris, T., and Pettingale, K. W., Psychological response to breast cancer: effect on outcome, *Lancet, 2,* 785-787, 1979.

Greer, S., Morris, T., Pettingale, K., and Haybittle, J., Mental attitudes to cancer: an additional prognostic factor, *Lancet,* 1, 750, 1985.

Grossarth-Maticek, R., Psychosocial predictors of cancer and internal diseases: an overview, *Psychother. Psychosom.,* 33, 122-128, 1980.

Guy, R., *An Essay On Schirrhous Tumours And Cancer,* W. Owen, London, 1759.

Hagnell, O., The premorbid personality of persons who develop cancer in a total population investigated in 1947 and 1957, *Ann. NY Acad. Sci.,* 125, 846-864, 1966.

Hall, H. R., Hypnosis and the immune system: a review with implications for cancer and the psychology of healing, *Am. J. Clin. Hypn.,* 25, 92-103, 1982.

Havlik, R. J., Vukasin, A. P., and Ariyan, S., The impact of stress on the clinical presentation of melanoma, *Piast. Reconstr. Surg., 90,* 57-61, 1992.

Hay, W. H., Cancer: A disease of either election or ignorance, *Am. J. Cancer,* 410-422, 1927.

Hedge, A. R., Hypnosis in cancer, *Br. J. Med. Hypn.,* 12, 2-5, 1960.

Heijnen, C. J., Kavelaars, A., and Ballieux, R., Corticotropin-releasing hormone and proopiomelanocortin-derived peptides in modulation of immune function, in *Psychoneuroimmunology,* 2nd ed., Ader, R., Felten, D. L., and Cohen, N., Eds., Academic Press, San Diego, CA, 1991, 429-446.

Helsing, K. J. and Szkło, M., Mortality after bereavement, *Am. J. Epidemiol.,* 114, 41-52, 1981.

Herbert, T. B. and Cohen, S., Stress and immunity in humans: a meta-ana- lytic review, *Ann. Behav. Med.,* 55, 364-379, 1993.

Holden, C., Cancer and the mind: how are they connected?, *Science,* 200, 1363-1368, 1978.

Holland, J. C., Behavioral and psychosocial risk factors in cancer: human studies, in Handbook of *Psychooncology,* Holland, J. C. and Rowland, J. H., Eds., Oxford University Press, New York, 1989, 612-627.

Holmes, T. H. and Rahe, R.H., The social readjustment rating scale, *J. Psychosom. Med.,* 11, 213-218, 1967.

Horrobin, D. F., Manku, M. S., Oka, M., Morgan, R. O., Cunnane, S. C., Ally, I., Ghayur, T., Schweitzer, M., and Karmali, R. A., The nutritional regulation of T lymphocyte function, *Med. Hypotheses,* 5, 969-985, 1979.

Ikeda, T. and Sirbasku, D. A., Purification and properties of a mammary- uterine pituitary tumor cell growth factor from pregnant sheep uterus, *Biol. Chem.,* 259, 4049-4064, 1984.

Ikemi, Y., Akagawa, S., Nakagawa, T., and Sugita, M., Psychosomatic considerations on cancer patients who have made a narrow escape from death, *Dynam. Psychiatry,* 31, 77-92, 1975.

Irwin, M. R., Hauger, R. L., Brown, M. R., and Britton, K. T., CRF activates autonomic nervous system and reduces natural killer cytotoxicity, *Am. J. Physiol.,* 255, R744-R747, 1988.

Irwin, M. R., Vale, W., and Britton, K. T., Central corticotropin-releasing factor suppresses natural killer cytotoxicity, *Brain Behav. Immun.,* 1, 81-87, 1987.

Irwin, M., Brain corticotropin-releasing hormone- and interleukin-1 beta- induced suppression of specific antibody production, *Endocrinology,* 133, 1352-1360, 1993.

Irwin, M., Daniels, M., Smith, T. L., Bloom, F., and Weiner, H., Impaired natural killer cell activity during bereavement, *Brain Behav. Immun.,* 1, 98-104, 1987.

Irwin, M., Hauger, R., and Brown, M., Central corticotropin-releasing hormone activates the sympathetic nervous system and reduces immune function: increased responsivity of the aged rat, *Endocrinology,* 131, 1047-1053, 1992.

Irwin, M., Patterson, T., Smith, T. L. et al., Reduction of immune function in life stress and depression, *Biol. Psychiatry,* 27, 22-30, 1990.

Jamison, R. N., Burish, T. G., and Wallston, K. A., Psychogenic factors in predicting survival of breast cancer patients, *J. Clin. Oncol.,* 5, 772-798, 1987.

Jenkins, C. D., Social environment and cancer mortality in men, *N. Engl. J. Med.,* 308, 395-398, 1983.

Johnson, H. M., Smith, E. M., Torres, B. A., and Blalock, J. E., Regulation of the *in vitro* antibody response by neuroendocrine hormones, *Proc. Natl. Acad. Sci. U.S.A.,* 79, 4171-4174, 1982.

Kakidani, H. et al., Cloning and sequence analysis of cDNA for porcine B- neo-endorphin/dymorphin precursor, *Nature,* 298, 245-249, 1982.

Kappas, A., Jones, H. E. H., and Roitt, I. M., Effects of steroid sex hormones on immunological phenomena, *Nature,* 198, 902, 1963.

Kegeles, S. S., Relationship of soc i ocu I tura Isociocultural factors to cancer, in *Cancer: The Behavioral Dimensions,* Cullen, J. W., Fox, B. H., and Isom, R. N., Eds., Raven Press, New York, 1976, 108-125.

Kiecolt-G laser, J. K., Glaser, R., Strain, E. C. et al., Modulation of cellular immunity in medical students, *J. Behav. Med., 9,* 5-21, 1986.

Kiecolt-Glaser, J. K. and Glaser, R., Stress and immune function in humans, in *Psychoneuroimmunoiogy,* 2nd ed., Ader, R., Felten, D. L., and Cohen, N., Eds., Academic Press, San Diego, CA., 1991, 849-867.

Kiecolt-Glaser, J. K., Garner, W., Speicher, C. et al., Psychosocial modifiers of immune competence in medical students, *Psychosom. Med.,* 46, 7-14, 1984.

Kissen, D. M., Brown, R. I. F., and Kissen, M. A., A further report on pers- onality and psychosocial factors in lung cancer, *Ann. NY Acad. Sci.,* 164, 535-545, 7969.

Kissen, D. M., Personality characteristics in males conducive to lung cancer, *Br. J. Med. Psychol.,* 36, 27-36, 1963.

Kissen, D. M., Psychosocial factors, personality and lung cancer, *Br. J. Med. Psychol.,* 40, 29-43, 1967.

Kissen, D. M., The significance of personality in lung cancer in men, *Ann. NY Acad. Sci.,* 125, 820-826, 1966.

Kissen, D., Psychosocial factors, personality and lung cancer in men aged 55-64, *Br. J. Med. Psychol.,* 40, 29-43, 1967.

Kissen, D., Psychosocial factors, personality and lung cancer in men aged 55-64, *Br. J. Med. Psychol.,* 40, 29-43, 1967.

Kissen, D., The present status of psychosomatic cancer research, *Geriatrics,* 24, 129, 1969.

Kneier, A. W. and Temoshok, L., Repressive coping reactions in patients with malignant melanoma as compared to cardiovascular patients, *J. Psychosom. Res., 28,* 145-155, 1984.

Kobasa, S., Maddi, S., and Kahn, S., Hardiness and health: a prospective study, *J. Personality Soc. Psychol.,* 42, 168-177, 1982.

Kronfol, Z., Silva, J., Greden, J., Dembiński, S., and Carroll, B. J., Cell-mediated immunity in melancholia, *Psychosom. Med.,* 44, 304, 1982.

Kune, G. A., Kune, S., and Watson, L. F., Perceived religiousness is protective for colorectal cancer: data from the Melbourne Colorectal Cancer Study, *J. R. Soc. Med.,* 86, 645-647, 1993.

Kune, G. A., Kune, S., Watson, L. F., and Bahnson, C. B., Personality as a risk factor in large bowel cancer: data from the Melbourne Colorectal Cancer Study, *Psychol. Med.,* 21, 29-41, 1991.

Kune, S., Kune, G. A., Watson, L. F., and Rahe, R. H., Recent life change and large bowel cancer: data from the Melbourne Colorectal Cancer Study, *J. Clin. Epidemiol.,* 44, 57-68, 1991.

Kune, S., Stressful life events and cancer, *Epidemiology, 4,* 395-397, 1993. Irwin, M., Daniels, M., and Weiner, H., Immune and neuroendocrine changes during bereavement, *Psychiatr. Clin. North Am.,* 10, 449-465, 1987.

Lambley, P., The role of psychological processes in the aetiology and treatment of cervical cancer: a biopsychological perspective, *Br. J. Med. Psychol.,* 66, 43-60, 1993.

Lapin, V., Pineal influences on tumor, *Prog. Brain Res.,* 52, 523-533, 1979. Dilman, V. M., Anisimov, V. N., Ostroumova, M. N., Morozov, V. G., Khavinson, V. K., and Azarova, M. A., Study of the anti-tumor effect of polvpeptide pineal extract, *Oncology,* 36, 274-280, 1979.

Le Shan, L. L. and Worthington, R. E., Personality as a factor in the pathogenesis of cancer, *Br. J. Mod. Psychol.,* 29, 49-56, 1956.

Le Shan, L., *You Can Fight For Your Life,* M. Evans, New York, 1977.

LeConte, J., Statistical researches on cancer, *South. Med Surg. J., 4,* 273-274, 1846.

Lehrer, S., Life change and gastric cancer, *Psychosom. Med.,* 42, 499-502, 1980.

Lehrer, S., Life change and lung cancer, J. *Hum. Stress,* 7, 7-11, 1981.

Lemonde, P., Influence of fighting on leukemia in mice, *Proc. Soc. Exp. Biol. Med.,* 102, 292-295, 1959.

LeShan, L. and Worthington, R. E., Some recurrent life history patterns observed in patients with malignant disease, *J. Nerv. Ment. Dis.,* 124, 460-465, 1956.

LeShan, L. L., An emotional life-history pattern associated with neoplastic disease, *Ann. NY Acad. Sci.,* 164, 546-557, 1969.

LeShan, L., Psychological states as factors in the development of malignant disease: a critical review, *J. Natl. Cancer Inst., 22,* 1-18, 1959.

Levenson, J. L. and Bernis, C., The role of psychological factors in cancer onset and progression, *Psychosomatics, 32,* 124-132, 1991.

Levitan, L. J., Levitan, H., and Levitan, M., The incidence of cancer in psychiatric patients: cancer and the emotions: a review, *Mt. Sinai J. Med., 41,* 627-631, 1980.

Levy, S. M., Herberman, R. B., Whiteside, T. et al., Perceived social support and tumor estrogen/progesterone receptor status as predictors of natural killer cell activity in breast cancer patients, *Psychosom. Med.,* 52, 73-85, 1990.

Levy, S., Herberman, R., Lippman, M. et al., Correlation of stress factors with sustained depression of natural killer cell activity and predicted prognosis in patients with breast cancer, *J. Clin. Oncol.,* 5, 348-353, 1987.

Levy, S., Herberman, R., Maluish, A. et al., Prognostic risk assessment in primary breast cancer by behavioral and immunological parameters, *Health Psychol.,* 4, 99-113, 1985.

Linn, B. S., Linn, M. W., and Jensen, J., Degree of depression and immune responsiveness, *Psychosom. Med.,* 44, 128-129, 1982.

Lippman, M. E., Endocrine responsive cancers in man, in *Textbook of Endocrinology,* Williams, R,, Ed., W. B. Saunders, Philadelphia, 1985, 286-302.

Lippman, M. E., Strobl, J., and Allegra, J. C., Effects of hormones in human breast cancers cells in tissue culture, in *Cell Biology of Breast Cancer,* McGrath, C., Brennan, M., and Rich, M., Eds., Academic Press, Orlando, FL, 1980, 218-234.

Lippman, M. E., Yarbro, G. K., and Leventhal, B. G., Effects of glucocorticoids on F_c receptors of a human granulocyte cell line, *Cancer Res.,* 38, 4251-4256, 1978.

Lippman, M. E., Yarbro, G. K., and Leventhal, B. G., Effects of glucocorticoids on F_c receptors of a human granulocyte cell line, *Cancer Research,* 38, 4251-4256, 1978.

Lippman, M. E., Yarbro, G. K., and Leventhal, B. G., Effects of glucocorticoids on F_c, receptors of a human granulocyte cell line, *Cancer Research,* 38, 4251-4256, 1978.

Marriott, D., Kirkwood, B. J., and Stough, C., Immunological effects of unemployment, *Lancet,* 344, 269-270, 1994.

McCruden, A. B. and Stimson, W. H., Sex hormones and immune function, in *Psychoneuroimmunology,* 2nd ed., Ader, R., Felten, D. L., and Cohen, N., Eds., Academic Press, San Diego, CA, 1991, 475-477.

Meares, A., A form of intensive meditation associated with the regression of cancer, *Am. J. Clin. Hypn.,* 25, 114-121, 1982.

Meares, A., Regression of cancer after intensive meditation, *Med. J. Aust., 2,* 184, 1976.

Meares, A., Regression of osteogenic sarcoma metastases associated with intensive meditation, *Med. J. Aust., 2,* 433, 1978.

Meares, A., Regression of recurrence of carcinoma of the breast at mastectomy site associated with intensive meditation, *Aust. Fam. Physician,* 10, 218-219, 1981.

Meares, A., Remission of massive metastasis from undifferentiated carcinoma of the lung associated with intensive meditation, *J. Am. Soc. Psychosom. Dent. Med., 21,* 40-41, 1980.

Meares, A., The quality of meditation effective in the regression of cancer, *J. Am. Soc. Psychosom. Dent. Med.,* 25, 129-132, 1978.

Meares, A., Vivid visualization and dim visual awareness in the regression of cancer in meditation, *J. Am. Soc. Psychosom. Dent. Med.,* 25, 85-88, 1978.

Miller, J., *Living Systems,* McGraw-Hill, New York, 1978.

Miller, T. and Spratt, J. S., Critical review of reported psychological correlates of cancer prognosis and growth, in *Mind and Cancer Prognosis,* Stoli, B. A., Ed., John Wiley & Sons, New York, 1979, 31-37.

Miller, T. R., Psychophysiologic aspects of cancer, *Cancer,* 39, 413, 1977.

Morris, T., Greer, S., Pettingale, K. W., and Watson, M., Patterns of expression of anger and their psychological correlates in women with breast cancer, *J. Psychosom. Res.,* 25, 111-117, 1981.

Morrison, F. R., Psychosocial factors in the etiology of cancer, *Diss. Abstr.Int., 42,* 155B, 1981.

Munck, A. and Guyre, P. M., Glucocorticoids and immune function, in *Psychoneuroimmunology,* 2nd ed., Ader, R., Felten, D. L., and Cohen, N., Eds., Academic Press, San Diego, CA, 1991, 447-460.

Nagy, E., Berczi, I., and Friesen, H. G., Regulation of immunity in rats by lactogenic and growth hormones, *Acta Endocrinol.,* 102, 351-357, 1983.

Nerozzi, D., Santoni, A., Bersani, G. et al., Reduced natural killer cell activity in major depression: neuroendocrine implications, *Psychoneuroendocrinoiogy,* 14, 295-301, 1989.

Nórdenstrom, B. E. W., Biologically Closed Electric Circuits: Clinical Experimental and Theoretical Evidence for an Additional Circulatory System, *Nordic Medical Publications, Stockholm, 1983, 358.*

Nórdenstrom, B. E., Impact of biologically closed electric circuits (BCEC) on structure and function, *Integr. Physiol. Behav. Sci.,* 27, 285-303, 1992.

Nunn, T. W., *On Cancer of the Breast, J* & A Churchill, London, 1882, 123.

Ogilvie, H., The human heritage, *Lancet,* ii, 42, 1957.

Osier, W., *Aequanimitas,* p. 258, McGraw-Hill, New York, 1906.

Osier, W., quoted in Lewison, E. F., Spontaneous regression of breast cancer, *Natl. Cancer Inst. Monogr.,* 44, 23, 1976.

Parry, C. H., quoted in Margetts, E. L., Historical notes on psychosomatic medicine, in *Recent Developments in Psychosomatic Medicine,* Vol. 1, Wittkower, E. D. and Cleghorn, R. A., Eds., Pitman and Sons, London, 1954, 56.

Pasteur, L., quoted in Selye, H., *The Stress of Life,* p. 205, McGraw-Hill, New York, 1956.

Pearson, H. A., Johnston, D., Smith, K. A., and Touloukian, R. J., The born- again spleen. Return of splenic function after splenectomy for trauma, *N. Engl. J. Med.,* 298, 1389-1392, 1978.

Pendergrass, E. P., Host resistance and other intangibles in the treatment of cancer, *Am. J. Roentgenol. Radium Ther.,* 85, 891, 1961.

Peters, L. J. and Mason, K. A., Influence of stress on experimental cancer, in *Mind and Cancer Prognosis,* Stoli, B. A., Ed., John Wiley & Sons, New York, 1979, 104-124.

Pettingale, K. W. and Hussein, M., Changes in immune status following conjugal bereavement, *StressMed.,* 10, 145-150, 1994.

Pettingale, K. W., Greer, S., and Tee, D. E. H., Serum IGA and emotional expression in breast cancer patients, *J. Psychosom. Res.,* 21, 395-399, 1977.

Pettingale, K. W., Towards a psychobiologic model of cancer: biological considerations, Soc. *Sci. Med., 20,* 779-787, 1985.

Pettingale, K. W., Watson, H., Tee, D. E. H., Inayat, Q., and Alhaq, A., A pathological grief, psychiatric symptoms and immune status following conjugal bereavement, *Stress Med.,* 5, 77-83, 1989.

Powell, C., *The Pathology of Cancer,* Macmillan, New York, 1908. Berglas, A., *Cancer: Its Nature, Cause and Cure,* Pasteur Institute Paris, 1957.

Pribram, K., Rethinking Neural Networks: Quantum Fields and Biological Data, *L. Erlbaum, New York, 1993.*

Renneker, R., Cancer and psychotherapy, in *Psychotherapeutic Treatment of Cancer Patients,* Goldberg, J., Ed., Free Press, New York, 1981, 131-166.

Riley, V., Cancer and stress: overview and critique, *Cancer Detection Prevention, 2,* 163-195, 1979.

Riley, V., Introduction: stress-cancer contradictions—a continuing puzzlement, *Cancer Detect. Prev., 2,* 159-162, 1979.

Riley, V., Mouse mammary tumors: alteration of incidence as apparent function of stress, *Science,* 189, 465-467, 1975.

Riley, V., Psychoneuroendocrine influences on immunocompetence and neoplasia, *Science,* 212, 1100-1109, 1981.

Roberts, M., *Malignancy and Evolution,* Grayson, New York, 1934. Moore, C. H., *The Antecedents of Cancer,* London, Longmans, 1865.

Rosch, P. J., Future directions in psychoneuroimmunology: psychoelectroneuro immunology?, in *Stress, the Immune System and Psychiatry,* Leonard, and Miller, K., Eds., John Wiley & Sons, Chichester, 1995.

Rosch, P. J., Growth and development of the stress concept and its significance in clinical medicine, in *Modern Trends in Endocrinology,* Hoeber, P. B., Ed., Butterworths, London, 1958, 278-297.

Rosch, P. J., Illness syndromes: high disability, in *Psychiatry in the Medical Specialties,* Dunbar, F., Ed., McGraw-Hill, New York, 1959, 152-317.

Rosch, P. J., Lifestyle and cancer, *NY State Med. J.,* 80, 2031-2038, 1980.

Rosch, P. J., Mind and cancer, *Lancet,* 1, 1302, 1979.

Rosch, P. J., Mind over cancer: some caveats, *StressMed.,* 10, 71, 1994.

Rosch, P. J., Ridiculous risk factors and heart attacks: diet-cholesterol dogma versus stress, *StressMed., 9,* 203-205, 1993.

Rosch, P. J., Some thoughts on the endemiology of cancer, *Cancer, Stress, and Death,* 2nd ed,, Day, S. B., Ed., Plenum Publishing, New York, 1986, 293-300.

Rosch, P. J., Some thoughts on the epidemiology of cancer, in *Readings in Oncology,* Day, S. B,, Sugarbaker, E. V, and Rosch, P. J., Eds. The International Foundation for Biosocial Development and Human Health, New York, 1980, 1-6.

Rosch, P. J., Stress and cancer, in *Psychosocial Stress and Cancer,* Cooper, C. L., Ed., John Wiley & Sons, London, 1984, 3-19.

Rosch, P. J., Stress and cancer: a disease of adaptation?, in *Cancer, Stress, and Death,* Tache, J., Selye, H., and Day, S. B., Eds., Plenum Publishing, New York, 1979, 187-212.

Rosch, P. J., Stress and electromedicine, *Med. Electron.,* 19(4), 124-128, 1989.

Rosch, P. J., Stress, cholesterol, and coronary heart disease, *Lancet,* ii, 851-852, 1983.

Rosch, P. J., Stress: cause or cure of cancer, in *Psychotherapeutic Treatment of Cancer Patients,* Goldberg, J., Ed., Free Press, New York, 1981, 39-57.

Rosch, P. J., Stress: its relationship with illness, in *Traumatic Medicine and Surgery For the Attorney,* III, part 6, Cantor, P.D., Ed., Butterworths, Washington, D.C, 1960, 261-364.

S. Keller, S. E. et al., Suppression of lymphocyte stimulation by anterior hypothalamic lesions in the guinea pig, *Cell. Immunol.,* 52, 334-340, 1980.

Salford, L. G., Persson, B. R., Brun, A., Ceberg, C. P., Kongstad, P. C., and Mir, L. M., A new brain tumor therapy combining bleomycin with in vivo electropermeabilization, *Biochem. Biophys. Res. Commun.,* 194, 938-943, 1993.

Sanyal, P. K., *History of Medicine and Pharmacy in India,* Amitava Sanyal, Calcutta, 1964.

Schleifer, S. J., Keller, S. E., Camerino, M. et al., Suppression of lymphocyte stimulation following bereavement, *JAMA,* 250, 374-377, 1983.

Schmale, A. H. and Iker, H. P., The affect of hopelessness and the development of cancer. I. The prediction of uterine cervical cancer in women with atypical cytology, *Psychosom. Med.,* 28, 714-721, 1966.

Schmale, A. H. and Iker, H. P., The affect of hopelessness and the development of cancer, *Psychosom. Med.,* 28, 714-721, 1966.

Schmale, A. H. and Iker, H. P., The psychological setting of uterine cervical Cancer, *Ann. NY Acad. Sci.,* 25, 807-813, 1966.

Schmale, A. H. and Iker, H., Hopelessness as a predictor of cervical cancer, *Soc. Sci. Med.,* 5, 95-100, 1971.

Schneider, J., *Stress, Loss and Grief,* University Park Press, Baltimore, 1984.

Schweitzer, A., *Forest Hospital of Lamborene,* Holt, Oxford, 1931. Stefansson, V., *Cancer: Disease of Civilization?,* Hill and Wang, New York 1960.

Seilerrn-Aspeng, F. and Kratochwil, K., Relation between regeneration and tumor growth, in *Regeneration in Animals and Related Problems,* Kioutsis, V. and Transpusch, H., Eds., North Holland, Amsterdam, 1965, 452-473.

Selye, H. and Rosch, P. J., Integration of endocrinology, in *Glandular Physiology and Therapy,* J. B. Lippincott, Philadelphia, 1946, 1-100.

Selye, H. and Rosch, P. J., The renaissance in endocrinology, in *Medicine and Science,* International University Press, New York, 1954, 30-49.

Selye, H., Foreword, in *Cancer, Stress, and Death,* Tache, J., Selye, H., and Day, B., Eds., Plenum Publishing, New York, 1979, xii.

Shaffer, J. W., Graves, P. L., Swank, R. T. et al., Clustering of personality traits in youth and the subsequent development of cancer among physicians, *J.Behav. Med.,* 10, 441-447, 1987.

Shamberger, R. J., Tytko, S. A., and Willis, C. E., Antioxidants in cereals and in food preservatives and declining cancer mortality, *Cleveland Clin. O.,* 39, 119-124, 1972.

Shekelle, R. B., Raynor, W. J., Ostfeld, A. M., Garron, D. C., Bieliauskas, L. A., Liu, S. C., Maliza, C., and Paul, O., Psychological depression and 17- year risk of death from cancer, *Psychosom. Med.,* 43, 117-125, 1981.

Sheldrake, R., *Rebirth of Nature,* Bantam, New York, 1992.

Snow, H., *Cancer and the Cancer Process,* Churchill, London, 1893. Kowal, S. J., Emotions as a cause of cancer: eighteenth and nineteenth century contributions, *Psychoanal. Rev.,* 42, 217-227, 1955.

Solve, H., Forty years of stress research: principal remaining problems and misconceptions, *Can. Med. Assoc. I.,* 115, 53-56, 1976.

Sontag, S., *Illness as Metaphor,* Farrar, Straus, and Giroux, New York, 1977.

Spiegel, D. and Sands, S. H., Psychological influences on metastatic disease progression, in *Progressive States of Malignant Neoplastic Growth,* Kaiser, H. E., Ed., Martinus Nijhoff, Dordrecht, The Netherlands, 1985, 74-89.

Spiegel, D., Bloom, J. R., and Yalom, I. D., Group support for patients with metastatic cancer: a randomized prospective outcome study, *Arch. Gen. Psychiatry,* 38, 527-533, 1981.

Spiegel, D., Bloom, J. R., Kraemer, H. C., and Gottheil, E., Effects of psychosocial treatment on survival of patients with metastatic breast cancer, *Lancet, 2,* 888-891, 1989.

Stein, M., Keller, S., and Schleifer, S., Role of the hypothalamus in mediating stress effects on the immune system, in *Mind and Cancer Prognosis,* Stoll, B. A., Ed., John Wiley & Sons, New York, 1979.

Stein, M., Miller, A. H., and Trestman, R. L., Depression, the immune system, and health and illness, *Arch. Gen. Psychiatry,* 48, 171-177, 1991.

Stein, M., Stress, brain and immune function, *Cerontologist, 22,* 203, 1982.

Stephenson, J. H. and Grace, W. J., Life stress and cancer of the cervix, *Psychosom. Med.,* 16, 287-294, 1954.

Stern, R., as quoted in Suess, R., Kinzel, V., and Scribner, J. P., *Cancer-Experiments and Concepts,* Springer-Verlag, New York, 1973.

Stroebe, W. and Stroebe, M. S., *Bereavement and Health,* Cambridge University Press, Cambridge, 1987.

Temoshok, L. and Dreher, H., *The Type C Connection: The Behavioral Links to Cancer and Your Health,* Penguin, New York, 1993.

Temoshok, L., Heller, B. W., and Sageviel, R. W. et al., The relationship of psychological factors of prognostic indicators in cutaneous malignant melanoma, *J. Psychosom. Res., 29,* 139-153, 1985.

Thomas, C. B. and Duszyński, K. R., Closeness to parents and the family constellation in a prospective study of five disease states: suicide, mental illness, malignant tumour, hypertension and coronary heart disease, *Johns Hopkins Med. J.,* 134, 251-270, 1974.

Thomas, C. B., Duszyński, K. R., and Shaffer, J. W., Family attitudes reported in youth as potential predictors of cancer, *Psychosom. Med.,* 41, 287-302, 1979.

Tolstoy, L., *The Death of Ivan llyitch,* Solotaroff, L., Ed., Bantam, New York, 1981.

Traue, H. C. and Pennebaker, J. W., *Emotion Inhibition and Health,* Hogrefe & Huber Publishers, Kirkland, WA, 1993.

Trichopoulos, D., MacMahon, B., and Brown, J., Socioeconomic status, urine estrogens, and breast cancer risk, *J. Natl. Cancer Inst.,* 64, 753-755, 1980.

Tromp, S. W., Meteorological stress and cancer, in *Stress and Cancer,* Bammer, K. and Newberry, B. H., Eds., C. J. Hogrefe, Toronto, 1981, 164-185.

Van Vollenhorn, R. F. and McGuire, J. L., Estrogen, progesterone and testosterone: can they be used to treat autoimmune disease?, *Cleveland Clin. J. Med.,* 61, 276-284, 1994.

Visintainer, M. A., Volpicelli, J. R., and Seligman, M. E. P., Tumor rejection in rats after inescapable or escapable shock, *Science,* 216, 437-439, 1982.

Walshe, W. H., *The Nature and Treatment of Cancer,* Taylor & Walton, London, 1846.

Warren, S. and Canavan, M. M., Frequency of cancer in the insane, *N. Engl. J. Med.,* 210, 739, 1934.

Wynder, E. L., Dietary habits and cancer epidemiology, *Cancer,* 43, 1955-1961, 1979.

Yamasaki, H., Aberrant expression and function of gap junctions during carcinogenesis, in *Nongenotoxic Mechanisms in Carcinogenesis,* Butterworth, B. E. and Slaga, T. J., Eds., Cold Spring Harbor Laboratory, Cold Spring Harbor, NY, 1987, 297-316.

Yirmiya, R., Shavit, Y., Ben-Eliyahu, S., Gale, R. P., Liebeskind, J. C., Taylor, A. N., and Weiner, H., Modulation of immunity and neoplasia by neuropeptides released by stressors, in *Stress, Neuropeptides, and Systemic Disease,* McCubbin, J. A., Kaufmann, P. G., and Nemeroff, C. B., Eds., Academic Press, San Diego, CA, 1991, 261-279.

Zagon, I. S. and McLaughlin, P. J., Endogenous opioid systems, stress and cancer, in *Enkephalins and Endorphins: Stress and the Immune System,* Plotnikoff, N. P., Faith, R. E., Murgo, A. J., and Good, R. A., Eds., Plenum, New York, 1986, 81-100.

Chapter IV

The Electrical Properties of Cancer Cells

About 100 years ago in the Western world, the study of biochemical interactions became the prevailing paradigm used to explain cellular functions and disease progression. The pharmaceutical industry subsequently became very successful in using this model in developing a series of effective drugs. As medicine became transformed into a huge business during the 20th century, medical treatments became largely based on drug therapies. These pharmaceutical successes have enabled pharmaceutical manufacturers to become wealthy and the dominant influence in medicine. At this point in time, the supremacy of the biochemical paradigm and pharmaceutical influences have caused almost all research in medicine to be directed toward understanding the chemistry of the body and the effects that patentable drugs have on altering that chemistry. Yet many biological questions cannot be answered with biochemical explanations alone, such as the role of endogenously-created electromagnetic fields and electrical currents in the body. In his book *Bioelectronics*, Albert Szent-Gyorgyi voiced his concern about some of the unanswered questions in biology: "No doubt, molecular biochemistry has harvested the greatest success and has given a solid foundation to biology. However, there are indications that it has overlooked major problems, if not a whole dimension, for some of the existing questions remain unanswered, if not unasked" (Szent-Gyorgyi, 1968). Szent-Gyorgyi believed that biochemical explanations alone fail to explain the role of electricity in cellular regulation. He believed that the cells of the body possess *electrical mechanisms* and use electricity to regulate and control the transduction of chemical energy and other life processes. Dr. Aleksandr Samuilovich Presman in his 1970 book *Electromagnetic Fields and Life* identified several significant effects of the interaction of electromagnetic fields with living organisms. Electromagnetic fields: 1) have information and communication roles in that they are employed by living organisms as information conveyors from the environment to the organism, within the organism and among organisms, and 2) are involved in life's vital processes in that they facilitate pattern formation, organization, and growth control within the organism (Presman, 1970). If living organisms possess the ability to utilize electromagnetic fields and electricity, there *must* exist physical structures within the cells that facilitate the sensing, transducing, storing, and transmitting of this form of energy.

Normal cells possess the ability to communicate information inside themselves and between other cells. The coordination of information by the cells of the body is involved in the regulation and integration of cellular functions and cell growth. When cancer arises, cancer cells are no longer regulated by the normal control mechanisms. When an injury occurs in the body, normal cells proliferate and replace the destroyed and damaged cells with either new cells or scar tissue. One characteristic feature of both proliferating cells and cancer cells is that these cells have cell membrane potentials that are lower than the cell membrane potential of healthy adult cells (Cone, 1975). After the repair is completed, the normal cells in the area of injury stop growing and their membrane potential returns to normal. In cancerous tissue, the electrical potential of cell membranes is maintained at a lower level than that of healthy cells and electrical connections are disrupted.

Cancerous cells also possess other features that are different from normal proliferating cells. Normal cells are well-organized in their growth, form strong contacts with their neighbors and stop growing when they repair the area of injury due to contact inhibition with other cells. Cancer cells are more easily detached and do not exhibit contact inhibition of their growth. Cancer cells become independent of normal tissue signaling and growth control mechanisms. In a sense, cancer cells have become desynchronized from the rest of the body. Examples of components that allow cells to function as solid-state electronic devices include: transducers (membrane receptors), inductors (membrane receptors and DNA), capacitors (cell and organelle membranes), resonators (membranes and DNA), tuning circuits (membrane-protein complexes), and semiconductors (liquid crystal protein polymers). The recognition that cancer cells have different electrical properties leads to therapies that address these electrical abnormalities and may have some benefit in cancer treatment.

Electricity, Charge Carriers, and Electrical Properties of Cells

The cells of the body are composed of matter. Matter itself is composed of atoms, which are mixtures of negatively charged electrons, positively charged protons, and electrically neutral neutrons.

Electric charges: When an electron is forced out of its orbit around the nucleus of an atom, the electron's action is known as electricity. An electron, an atom, or a material with an excess of electrons has a negative charge. An atom or a substance with a deficiency of electrons has a positive charge. Like charges repel, while unlike charges attract.

Electrical potentials are created in biological structures when charges are separated. A material with an electrical potential possesses the capacity to do work.

Electric field: "An electric field forms around any electric charge" (Becker, 1985). The potential difference between two points produces an electric field represented by electric lines of flux. The negative pole always has more electrons than the positive pole. Electricity is the flow of mobile charge carriers in a conductor or a semiconductor from areas of high charge to areas of low charge driven by the electrical force. Any machinery, whether it is mechanical or biological, that possesses the ability to harness this electrical force has the ability to do work.

Voltage also depends on this potential difference or electromotive force. A current will not flow unless it gets a push. When two areas of unequal charge are connected, a current will flow in an attempt to equalize the charge difference. The difference in potential between two points gives rise to a voltage, which causes charge carriers to move and current to flow when the points are connected. This force cause motion and causes work to be done.

Current is the rate of flow of charge carriers in a substance past a point. The unit of measure is the ampere. In inorganic materials, electrons carry the current. In biological tissues, both mobile ions and electrons carry currents. In order to make electrical currents flow, a potential difference must exist and the excess electrons on the negatively charged material will be pulled toward the positively charged material. A flowing electric current always produces an expanding magnetic field with lines of force at a 90-degree angle to the direction of current flow. When a current increases or decreases, the magnetic field strength increases or decreases the same way.

Conductor - in electrical terms, a conductor is a material in which the electrons are mobile.

An *insulator* is a material that has very few free electrons.

A *semiconductor* is a material that has properties of both insulators and conductors. In general, semiconductors conduct electricity in one direction better than they will in the other direction. Semiconductors can functions as conductors or as insulators, depending on the direction the current is flowing.

Resistance – No materials, whether they are non-biological or biological, will perfectly conduct electricity. All materials will resist the flow of an electric charge through it, causing a dissipation of energy as heat. Resistance is measured in ohms, according to Ohm's law. In simple DC circuits, resistance equals impedance.

Impedance denotes the relation between the voltage and the current in a component or system. Impedance is usually described "as the opposition to the flow of an alternating electric current through a conductor. However, impedance is a broader concept that includes the phase shift between the voltage and the current" (Ivorra, 2002).

Inductance – The expansion or contraction of a magnetic field varies as the current varies and causes an electromotive force of self-induction, which opposes any further change in the current. Coils have greater inductance than straight conductors so in electronic terms, coils are called inductors. When a conductor is coiled, the magnetic field produced by current flow expands across adjacent coil turns. When the current changes, the induced magnetic field that is created also changes and creates a force called the counter emf that opposes changes in the current. This effect does not occur in static conditions in DC circuits when the current is steady. The effect only arises in a DC circuit when the current experiences a change in value. When current flow in a DC circuit rapidly falls, the magnetic field also rapidly collapses and has the capability of generating a high induced emf that at times can be many times the original source voltage. Higher induced voltages may be created in an inductive circuit by increasing the speed of current changes and increasing the number of coils. In alternating current (AC) circuits, the current continuously changes so that the induced emf will affect current flow at all times. *We should interject at this point that a number of membrane proteins as well as DNA consist of helical coils, which may allow them to electronically function as inductor coils. Also, some research that we have seen also indicates that biological tissues may possess superconducting properties. If certain membrane proteins and the DNA actually function as electrical inductors, they may enable the cell to transiently produce very high electrical voltages.*

Capacitance is the ability to accumulate and store charge from a circuit and later give it back to a circuit. In DC circuits, capacitance opposes any change in circuit voltage. In a simple DC circuit, current flow stops when a capacitor becomes charged. Capacitance is defined by the measure of the quantity of charge that has to be moved across the membrane to produce a unit change in membrane potential.

Capacitors in electrical equipment are composed of two plates of conducting metals that sandwich an insulating material. Energy is taken from a circuit to supply and store charge on the plates. Energy is returned to the circuit when the charge is removed. The area of the plates, the amount of plate separation, and the type of dielectric material used all affect the capacitance. The dielectric characteristics of a material include both conductive and capacitive properties (Reilly, 1998). In cells, the cell membrane is a leaky dielectric. *This means that any condition, illness, or change in dietary intake that affects the composition of the cell membranes and their associated minerals can affect and alter cellular capacitance.* Inductors in electronic equipment exist in series and in parallel with other inductors as well as with resistors and capacitors. Resistors slow down the rate of conductance by brute force. Inductors impede the flow of electrical charges by temporarily *storing energy as a magnetic field* that gives back the energy later. Capacitors impede the flow of electric current by *storing the energy as an electric field.* Capacitance becomes an important electrical property in AC circuits and pulsating DC circuits. The tissues of the body contain pulsating DC circuits (Becker and Selden, 1985) and AC electric fields (Liboff, 1997). Cellular electrical properties, electromagnetic fields (EMF), and EMF effects on cells will be discussed in later sections of this monograph. These effects include: ligand receptor interactions of hormones, growth factors, cytokines, and neurotransmitters leading to alteration/initiation of membrane regulation of internal cellular processes, alteration of mineral entry through the cell membrane, activation or inhibition of cytoplasmic enzyme reactions, increasing the electrical potential and capacitance of the cell membrane, changes in dipole orientation, activation of the DNA helix by untwisting the helix leading to increased reading and transcription of codons and an increase in protein synthesis, activation of cell membrane receptors that act within certain windows of frequency and amplitude leading to the concepts of electromagnetic reception, transduction, and attunement.

In order to understand how weak EMFs have biological effects, it is important to understand certain concepts, including the following: electric fields need to be measured not just as strong or weak, but also as low carriers or high carriers of information. This is because electric fields conventionally-defined as thermally-strong may be low in biological information content and electric fields conventionally-considered as thermally-weak or non-ionizing may be high in biological information content if the proper receiving equipment exists in biological tissues. Weak electromagnetic fields include bioenergetic, bioinformational, non-ionizing, and non-thermal, while each exerts measurable biological effects. Weak electromagnetic fields have effects on biological organisms, tissues, and cells that are highly frequency-specific and the dose response curve is non-linear. Because the effects of weak electromagnetic fields are non-linear, fields in the proper frequency and amplitude windows may produce large effects, which may be beneficial or harmful. Homeopathy is an example of a weak field with a beneficial electromagnetic effect. Examples of thermally weak fields with high information content of the right frequency range are visible light and healing touch.

Biological tissues have electronic components that can receive, transduce, and transmit weak electronic signals that are actually below thermal noise.

Biological organisms use weak electromagnetic fields (electric and photonic) to communicate with all parts of themselves. An electric field can carry information through frequency and amplitude fluctuations. Healthy biological organisms have coherent biofields while unhealthy organisms have field disruptions and unintegrated signals. Corrective measures to correct field disruptions and improve field integration such as acupuncture, neural therapy, and resonant repatterning therapy promote health.

More Details about the Electrical Roles of Membranes and Mitochondria

Electricity in the body comes from the food that we eat and the air that we breathe (Brown, 1999). Cells derive their energy from enzyme-catalyzed chemical reactions, which involves the oxidation of fats, proteins, and carbohydrates. Cells can produce energy by oxygen-dependent aerobic enzyme pathways and by less efficient fermentation pathways. The specialized proteins and enzymes involved in oxidative phosphorylation are located on the inner mitochondrial membrane and form a molecular respiratory chain or wire. This molecular wire (electron transport chain) passes electrons donated by several important electron donors through a series of intermediate compounds to molecular oxygen, which becomes reduced to water. In the process, ADP is converted into ATP. When the electron donors of the respiratory chain NADH and FADH2 release their electrons, hydrogen ions are also released. These positively-charged hydrogen ions are pumped out of the mitochondrial matrix across the inner mitochondrial membrane creating an electrochemical gradient. At the last stage of the respiratory chain, these hydrogen ions are allowed to flow back across the inner mitochondrial membrane and they drive a molecular motor called ATP synthase in the creation of ATP, like water drives a water wheel (Stipanuk, 2000). *This normal energy production process utilizing electron transport and hydrogen ion gradients across the mitochondrial membrane is disrupted when cells become cancerous. What structures are involved in cancerous transformation?* Many current cancer researchers believe that cancerous transformation arises due to changes in the genetic code. However, more seems to be happening in these cases than genetic abnormalities alone. A series of papers written by Ilmensee, Mintz, and Hoppe in the 1970-1980s showed that replacing the fertilized nucleus of a mouse ovum by the nucleus of a teratocarcinoma did not create a mouse with cancer. Instead, the mice were born cancer-free (Seeger and Wolz, 1990). These studies support the theory that abnormalities in other cell structures outside of the nucleus, such as the cell membrane and the mitochondria, and functional disturbances in cellular energy production and cell membrane potential are also involved in cancerous transformation. As far back as 1938, Dr. Paul Gerhardt Seeger originated the idea that destruction or inactivation of enzymes, like cytochrome oxidase, in the respiratory chain of the mitochondria was involved in the development of cancer. Seeger indicated in his publications that the initiation of malignant degeneration was due to alterations not to the nucleus, but to cytoplasmic organelles (Seeger and Wolz, 1990).

Mitochondrial dysfunction and changes in cytochrome oxidase have also been reported by other cancer researchers (Sharp et al., 1992; Modica-Napolitano et al., 2001). Seeger's findings after over 50 years of cancer research are that cells become more electronegative in the course of cancerization, that *membrane degeneration* occurs in the initial phase of carcinogenesis first in the external cell membrane and then in the inner mitochondrial membrane, that the degenerative changes in the surface membrane cause these *membranes to become more permeable to water-soluble substances* so that potassium, magnesium, and calcium migrate from the cells and sodium and water accumulate in the cell interior, that the degenerative changes in the inner membrane of the mitochondria causes *loss of anchorage of critical mitochondrial enzymes*, and that the mitochondria in cancer cells degenerate and are reduced in number (Seeger and Wolz, 1990). Numerous toxins have been identified that are capable of causing cancerous transformation. Many toxins not only cause genetic abnormalities, but also affect the structure and function of the cell membrane and the mitochondria. Toxic compounds that disrupt the electrical potential of cell membranes and the structure of mitochondrial membranes will deactivate the electron transport chain and disturb oxygen-dependent energy production. Cells will then revert to fermentation, which is a less efficient primeval form of energy production. According to Seeger, the conversion to glycolysis secondary to the deactivation of the electron transport chain has a profound effect on the proliferation of tumor cells. Seeger believes that the virulence of cancer cells is inversely proportional to the activity of the respiratory chain. Conversion to glycolysis as a primary mechanism for energy production results in excessive accumulation of organic acids and pH alterations in cancerous tissues (Seeger and Wolz, 1990). The body is an electrical machine and the matrix of cells that compose the body possess electrical properties. Among the electrical properties that cells manifest are the ability to conduct electricity, create electrical fields, and function as electrical generators and batteries. This sounds like the basis of a good science fiction movie. In electrical equipment, the electrical charge carriers are electrons. In the body, electricity is carried by a number of mobile charge carriers as well as electrons. Although many authorities would argue that electricity in the body is only carried by charged ions, Robert O. Becker and others have shown that electron semiconduction also takes place in biological polymers (Becker and Selden, 1985; Becker, 1990). The major charge carriers of biological organisms are negatively-charged electrons, positively-charged hydrogen protons, positively-charged sodium, potassium, calcium, and magnesium ions and negatively-charged anions, particularly phosphate ions. The work of Mae Wan Ho and Fritz Popp indicate that cells and tissues also conduct and are linked by electromagnetic phonons and photons (Ho, 1996). The body uses the exterior cell membrane and positively-charged mineral ions that are maintained in different concentrations on each side of the cell membrane to create a cell membrane potential (a voltage difference across the membrane) and a strong electrical field around the cell membrane. This electrical field is a readily-available source of energy for a significant number of cellular activities including membrane transport, and the generation of electrical impulses in the brain, nerves, heart, and muscles (Brown, 1999). The storage of electrical charge in the membrane and the generation of an electrical field create a battery function so that the liquid crystal semiconducting cytoskeletal proteins can, in a sense, plug into this field and powered-up cell structures such as genetic material. The voltage potential across the membrane creates a surprisingly powerful electric field that is 10,000,000 volts/meter according to Reilly and up to 20,000,000 volts/meter according to Brown (Reilly, 1998; Brown, 1999). The body uses the mitochondrial membrane and positively-charged hydrogen ions to create a strong membrane potential across the mitochondrial membrane. Hydrogen ions are maintained in a high concentration of the outside of the mitochondrial membrane by the action of the electron transport chain, which creates a mitochondrial membrane potential of about 40,000,000 volts/meter. When this proton electricity flows back across the inner mitochondrial membrane, it is used to power a molecular motor called ATP synthase, which loads negatively charged phosphate anions onto ADP, thus creating ATP (Brown, 1999). ADP, ATP, and other molecules that are phosphate carriers are electrochemical molecules that exchange phosphate charges between other cellular molecules. According to Brown, "The flow of phosphate charge is not used to produce large-scale electrical gradients, as in conventional electricity, but rather more local electrical field within molecules" (Brown, 1999). The body uses phosphate electricity to activate and deactivate enzymes in the body by charge transfer, which causes these enzymes to switch back and forth between different conformational states. So in a sense, enzymes and other types of proteins, such as cytoskeletal proteins, may function as electrical switches. The liquid crystal proteins that compose the cytoskeleton support stabilize and connect the liquid crystal components of the cell membrane with other cell organelles. The cytoskeletal proteins have multiple roles. The proteins that compose the cytoskeleton serve as *mechanical scaffolds* that organize enzymes and water, and anchor the cell to structures in the extracellular matrix via linkages through the cell membrane (Wolfe, 1993). According to Wolfe, "Cytoskeletal frameworks also reinforce the plasma membrane and fix the positions of junctions, receptors, and connections to the extracellular matrix" (Wolfe, 1993).

Self-assembling cytoskeletal proteins are dynamic network structures that create a fully-integrated electronic and probably fiberoptic *continuum* that links and integrates the proteins of the extracellular matrix with the cell organelles (Haltiwanger, 1998; Oschman, 2000).

Cytoskeletal proteins also structurally- and electronically-link the cell membrane to cell organelles. Cytoskeletal proteins are altered in cancer cells. Alterations include: *reversion to arrangements typical of embryonic cells* and breakage of contact and connections with ECM and neighboring cells. *It is our opinion that change of connections of the cytoskeletal proteins with ECM components and the cell membrane will disrupt the flow of inward current into the cell, affect genetic activity, and is an important factor in disabling oxygen-dependent energy production.* Cells can obtain energy from food either by fermentation or oxygen-mediated cellular respiration. Both methods start with the process of glycolysis, which is the splitting of glucose (6 carbon) into two molecules of pyruvate (3 carbon). Most biologists believe that glycolysis, the oldest metabolic way to produce ATP, has been conserved in all living organisms. Glycolysis happens in the cytoplasm and does not require oxygen in order to produce ATP, but it is also a much less efficient method than aerobic respiration. The enzyme pyruvate dehydrogenase occupies a pivotal role in determining whether energy is extracted from glucose by aerobic or anaerobic methods (Garnett, 1998). This enzyme exists in an altered form in cancer cells (Garnett, 1998). *Over all membrane changes, mitochondrial dysfunction, loss of normal cellular electronic connections, and enzyme changes are all factors that contribute to the permanent reliance of cancer cells on glycolysis for energy production.* The electronic roles of the cell membrane and the electrical charge of cell surface coats in include cell membrane potential. All cells possess an electrical potential (a membrane potential) that exists across the cell membrane. Why is this so? Cell membranes are composed of a bilayer of highly mobile lipid molecules that electrically act as an insulator (dielectric). The insulating properties of the cell membrane lipids also act to restrict the movement of charged ions and electrons across the membrane except through specialized membrane-spanning protein ion channels (Aidley and Stanfield, 1996) and membrane-spanning protein semiconductors (Oschman, 2000).

Because the cell membrane is selectively-permeable to sodium and potassium ions, a different concentration of these and other charged mineral ions will build up on either side of the membrane. The different concentrations of these charged molecules cause the outer membrane surface to have a relatively higher positive charge than the inner membrane surface and creates an electrical potential across the membrane (Charman, 1996). All cells have an imbalance in *electrical charges* between the inside of the cell and the outside of the cell. The difference is known as the membrane potential. Because the membrane potential is created by the difference in the concentration of ions inside and outside the cell, this creates an electrochemical force across the cell membrane (Reilly, 1998). "Electrochemical forces across the membrane *regulate chemical exchange across the cell*" (Reilly, 1998). The cell membrane potential helps control cell membrane permeability to a variety of nutrients and helps turn on the machinery of the cell, particularly energy production and the synthesis of macromolecules. All healthy living cells have a membrane potential of about -60 to –100mV. The negative sign of the membrane potential indicates that the inside surface of the cell membrane is relatively more negative than the immediate exterior surface of the cell membrane (Cure, 1991). In a healthy cell, the inside surface of the cell membrane is slightly negative relative to its external cell membrane surface (Reilly, 1998). When one considers the transmembrane potential of a healthy cell, the electric field across the cell membrane is enormous – up to 10,000,000 to 20,000,000 volts/meter (Reilly, 1998; Brown, 1999). Healthy cells maintain, inside of themselves, a high concentration of potassium and a low concentration of sodium. But when cells are injured or cancerous sodium and water flows in to the cells, potassium, magnesium, calcium, and zinc are lost from the cell interior and the cell membrane potential falls (Cone, 1970, 1975, 1985; Cope, 1978). It is known that cancer changes cell membrane structure, membrane function, concentrations of minerals in cells, cell membrane potential, the electrical connections within the cells and between cells, and cellular energy production.

Cells actually have a number of discrete electrical zones. According to Charman, a cell contains four electrified zones (Charman, 1996). The *central zone* contains negatively-charged organic molecules and maintains a steady bulk negativity. An *inner positive zone* exists between the inner aspect of the cell membrane and the central negative zone. The inner positive zone is composed of a thin layer of freely mobile mineral cations, particularly potassium and, according to Hans Nieper (Nieper, 1985), a small amount of calcium as well. The *outer positive zone* exists around the outer surface of the cell membrane and consists of a denser zone of mobile cations composed mostly of sodium, calcium, and a small amount of potassium. Because the concentration of positive charges is larger on the outer surface of the cell membrane than the concentration of positive charges on the inner surface of the cell membrane, an electrical potential exists across the cell membrane. One might ask at this point how the surface of cells can be electrically-negative if a shell of positively-charged mineral ions surrounds the exterior surface of the cell membrane. The answer lies in the existence of an outer electrically-negative zone composed of the glycocalyx.

The *outermost electrically-negative zone* is composed of negatively-charged sialic acid molecules that cap the tips of glycoproteins and glycolipids that extend outward from the cell membrane like tree branches. The outermost negative zone is separated from the positive cell membrane surface by a distance of about 20 micrometers. According to Charman, "It is this outermost calyx zone of steady negativity that makes each cell act as a negatively charged body; every cell creates a negatively charged field around itself that influences any other charged body close to it" (Charman, 1996). It is the negatively-charged sialic acid residue of the cell coat (glycocalyx) that gives each cell its zeta potential. Since the negatively-charged electric fields around cells are created by sialic acid residues, any factor that increases or decreases the number of sialic acid residues will change the degree of surface negativity a cell exhibits. We will discuss later in this chapter how cancer cells have significantly more sialic acid molecules in their cell coat and, as a result, cancer cells have a greater surface negativity. *In our opinion, one of reasons that enzyme therapy is beneficial in cancer is because certain enzymes can remove sialic acid residues from cancer cells, reducing their surface negativity.*

The Electrical Properties of Cancer Cells, Part 1

Some of the characteristic features of cancerous cells that affect their electrical activity are: 1) Cancer cells are less efficient in their production of cellular energy (ATP), 2) Cancer cells have cell membranes that exhibit different electrochemical properties and a different distribution of electrical charges than normal tissues (Cure, 1991, 1995; Revici, 1961), 3) Cancer cells have altered membrane composition and membrane permeability, which results in the movement of potassium, magnesium, and calcium out of the cell and the accumulation of sodium and water into the cell (Seeger and Wolz, 1990), and 4) Cancer cells have lower potassium concentrations and higher sodium and water content than normal cells (Cone, 1970, 1975; Cope, 1978). The result of these mineral movements, membrane composition changes, energy abnormalities, and membrane charge distribution abnormalities is a drop in the normal membrane potential and membrane capacitance. We will now discuss these features in more depth. One of the characteristic features of injured and cancerous cells is that they are less efficient in their production of cellular energy (ATP). One of the mysteries of cancer is whether energy abnormalities cause or contribute to the mineral alterations or whether mineral alterations and membrane changes cause or contribute to the energy abnormalities by disrupting mitochondrial production of ATP. But all these abnormalities are present and, in our opinion, all of them should be addressed by therapeutic strategies. A *change in mineral content of the cell,* particularly an increase in the intracellular concentration of positively-charged sodium ions and an *increase in negative charges on the cell coat* (glycocalyx), are two of the major factors causing cancerous cells to have lower membrane potential than healthy cells (Cure, 1991). Cancer cells exhibit both *lower electrical membrane potentials and lower electrical impedance* than normal cells (Cone, 1985; Blad and Baldetorp, 1996; Stern, 1999). Since the membrane potential in a cancer cell is consistently weaker than the membrane potential of a healthy cell, the electrical field across the membrane of a cancer cell will be reduced. The reduction in membrane electrical field strength will, in turn, cause alterations in the metabolic functions of the cell. In the resting phase, normal cells maintain a high membrane potential of around -60mv to -100mv, but when cells begin cell division and DNA synthesis, the membrane potential falls to around -15mv (Cure, 1995). When a cell has completed cell division, its membrane potential will return back to normal. According to Cone, two of the most outstanding electrical features of cancer cells are that they constantly maintain their membrane potential at *a low value* and their intracellular *concentration of sodium at a high concentration* (Cone, 1970, 1975, 1985). Cone has discussed in his publications that a sustained elevation of intracellular sodium may act as a mitotic trigger, causing cells to go into cell division (mitosis) (Cone, 1985). It is generally thought that a *steady supply of cellular energy* and a healthy cell membrane are needed to maintain a normal or healthy concentration of intracellular minerals and a healthy membrane potential. This means that conditions associated with disruption of cellular energy production and membrane structure/function will result in *changes in the intracellular mineral concentration and a low membrane potential.* This statement may be true for injured cells, but Cure has proposed that another additional factor may be involved in changing the cell membrane potential of cancer cells, the concentration of sodium and potassium inside of cancer cells, and the mechanisms that cancer cells use to produce energy. Cure has proposed that the accumulation of an excessive amount of negative charges on the exterior surface of cancer cells will depolarize cancer cell membranes. He thinks that the depolarization (fall in membrane potential) of the cancer cell membrane due to the accumulation of excess negative surface charges may precede and create the reduction in intracellular potassium and the rise in the intracellular sodium launching the cell into a carcinogenic state (Cure, 1991). We know this must read like we am splitting hairs, but if the creation of an excessive negative charge on the surface of a cell can initiate a carcinogenic change, then it means genetic changes can result from the development of cellular electrical abnormalities. This has profound implications because it would mean that the development of genetic abnormalities is not always the prime factor leading to cancerous transformation. Cure's theory ties into Dr. Paul Gerhardt Seeger's work that cancer arises from alterations in the functions of cell organelles outside of the nucleus (Seeger and Wolz, 1990). This idea may mean that certain chemicals, viruses, and bacteria create cancers by modifying the electrical charge of the cell surface, resulting in alterations in cell membrane and organelle membrane electrical potentials, the functions of these membranes, intracellular mineral content, energy production, and genetic expression. It also means that therapeutic methods that manipulate the electrical charge of cell membranes, the composition of cell membranes, and the content of intracellular minerals can result in alterations in genetic activity. A healthy cell membrane potential is strongly linked to the control of cell membrane transport mechanisms as well as DNA activity, protein synthesis, and aerobic energy production. Since injured and cancerous cells cannot maintain a normal membrane potential, they will have electronic dysfunctions that will impede repair and the reestablishment of normal metabolic functions. Therefore, a key component of cell repair and cancer treatment would be to reestablish a healthy membrane potential in the body's cells (Nieper, 1966a, 1966b, 1966c, 1967a, 1967b, 1968, 1985; Alexander, 1997b; Nieper et al., 1999).

The Electrical Properties of Cancer Cells, Part 2

The idea of classifying cancers by their electrical properties is not a new idea – in fact, it was first proposed by Fricke and Morse in 1926 (Fricke and Morse, 1926). For example, the electrical conductivity and permittivity of cancerous tissue has been found to be greater than the electrical conductivity and permittivity of normal tissues (Foster and Schepps, 1981). Because cancerous cells demonstrate greater permittivity, which is the ability to resist the formation of an electrical field, they will resonate differently from normal cells.

The electrical conductivity of a tissue depends on both the physico-chemical bulk properties – i.e., properties of tissue fluids and solids – and the microstructural properties – i.e., the geometry of microscopic compartments (Scharfetter, 1999). In turn, the electrical conductivity and permittivity of biological materials will vary characteristically, *depending on the frequency applied* (Scharfetter, 1999).

In biological tissues, electrical currents are carried by both ionic conduction and electron semiconduction. Whereas in electrical equipment, only electrons or electron holes carry the electrical current. Therefore, the electrical properties of biological tissues are dependent on all the physical mechanisms, which control the mobility and availability of the relevant ions, such as sodium, chloride, potassium, magnesium, and calcium (Scharfetter, 1999). The electrical charges associated with semiconducting proteins and extracellular matrix proteoglycans also contribute to the conductivity of a tissue. So the electrical properties of tissues also relate to electron availability, which can be affected by such factors as the degree of tissue acidity, the degree of tissue hypoxia, the degree that water is structured, and the availability of electron donors such as antioxidants, and the presence of electrophilic compounds on the cell membrane and in the extracellular matrix (ECM). The cell membrane ECM interface is the location where molecules like hormones, peptide growth factors, cytokines, and neurotransmitters initiate chemical signaling from cell to cell and where these chemical-signaling events can be regulated and amplified by the weak non-ionizing oscillating electromagnetic fields that are naturally present in the ECM (Adey, 1988). The cell membrane ECM interface has a lower electrical resistance than the cell membrane so *electrical currents will be preferentially conducted* through this space (Adey, 1981). This cell surface current flow is involved in controlling many of the physiological functions of the cells and tissues (Adey, 1981). Conductivity in both healthy tissues and cancerous tissues can be affected by variations in temperature, oxygen levels, mineral concentrations in intracellular and extracellular fluid, the types of minerals present in intracellular and extracellular fluids, pH (both intracellular and extracellular), level of hydration (cell water content and extracellular water content), the ratio of structured/unstructured water inside of the cell, membrane lipid/sterol composition, free radical activity, the amount of negative charges present on the surface of cell membranes, the amount and structure of hyaluronic acid in the

ECM, the emergence of endogenous electrical fields, the application of external electromagnetic fields, and the presence of chemical electrophilic toxins and heavy metals both within the cell and in the ECM. According to Dr. Robert Pekar, "Every biological process is also an electric process" and "health and sickness are related to the bio-electric currents in our body" (Pekar, 1997). The electrical properties of cancer cells are different than the electrical properties of the normal tissues that surround them. From the papers that we have read in preparing this monograph, many authors have reported that cancer cells have higher intracellular sodium, higher content of unstructured water, lower intracellular potassium, magnesium and calcium concentrations, and more negative charges on their cell surface (Hazelwood et al., 1974; Cone, 1975; Cope, 1978; Brewer, 1985, Cure, 1991). These abnormalities result in cancer cells having lower transmembrane potentials than normal cells and altered membrane permeability. These cell membrane changes interfere with the flow of oxygen and nutrients into the cells and impair aerobic metabolism causing cancer cells to rely more on anaerobic metabolism for energy production. Anaerobic metabolism, excessive sodium concentrations, low transmembrane potential, and pH alterations in turn create intracellular conditions more conducive to cellular mitosis. Recognizing that cancer cells have altered electrical properties also leads to strategies toward correcting these properties.

Manipulation of fatty acids and sterols to address membrane composition. There is a search to find methods to reduce intracellular sodium concentrations, since an intracellular excess of positively-charged sodium ions reduces the negative interior potential of the inner membrane surface, resulting in a fall in membrane potential.

Manipulating electrical charges on both sides of tumor cell membranes. Corrective intracellular, extracellular, and membrane measures can be used to address the abnormal electrical properties of cancer cells. Intracellular measures could include the use of intracellular potassium and magnesium mineral transporters and the amino acid taurine to reestablish more normal intracellular levels of these minerals inside of the cell. Calcium aspartate can be used to deposit calcium on the inner side of the cell membrane. Extracellular measures could include the use of calcium 2-AEP to lay down a shell of positive calcium ions on the surface of cells to neutralize the negative surface charges. Also, enzymes and antihCG vaccines can reduce the number of negatively-charged sialic acid residues on the surface of cancer cells. Cell membrane measures could include the use of squalene to improve sodium excretion from the cell and oxygen entry into the cells. In summary, improved cell membrane potential and membrane capacitance will affect mitochondrial production of ATP, cell membrane permeability, and the production of proteins and other macromolecules. Certain nutrients have the ability to support the electrical potential of the cell membrane. These nutrients include essential fatty acids, phospholipids, sterols, and nutrients such as mineral transporters that help normalize intracellular mineral concentrations in diseased cells. The combination of cell membrane repair and correction of deficiencies of intracellular mineral concentrations, primarily potassium, magnesium, zinc, and calcium, and correction of excessive intracellular levels of sodium will result in improvement of cell membrane capacitance back toward a healthier charge. Mineral transporters such as orotates, arginates, and aspartates can be used to adjust intracellular mineral concentrations. Some clinicians also try to improve the cellular capacitance of cancer cells through the use of PEMF, microcurrent, infrared, and phototherapy equipment. Tissue cells exist within a continuum where they are attached to other cells of the same type. The cells of the body require a steady supply of nutrients so they are typically located in close proximity to blood vessels. The extracellular matrix occupies an intermediate position between the blood vessels and the cell membrane. The major anatomical areas we will examine are:

1. The intravascular space and its components
2. The cell membrane covering of cells and the attached glycocalyx
3. The extracellular space and the components of the extracellular matrix
4. The ECM-glycocalyx-membrane interface

The intravascular space and its components have many functions, including nutrient transport into the cell, toxin transport away from the cells, and a control function where soluble hormones, growth stimulants, and inhibitors are carried to cells from distant locations and away from secreting cells to distant locations.

Chemical and anatomical roles of the cell membrane. The cell membrane is the gatekeeper of the cell that controls the inflow and outflow of nutrients and electric currents to and from the cell interior. It regulates the active transport of nutrients such as minerals and amino acids, and the release of toxins. The cell membrane is an interface between the cell interior, other cells, and components of the extracellular matrix (ECM). The cell membrane mediates adherence and communication with other cells, the ECM, and components of the immune system. Normal multicellular organisms require coherent and coordinated communication of each cell with the other cells in the organism. In order to synchronize cellular processes in a multicellular state, *a communication system must exist*. For most of the last century, biological science has concentrated almost exclusively on explaining the communication system of multicellular organisms with vascular systems by focusing on circulatory chemical signals carried by the bloodstream to other areas of the body. This paradigm attributes communication at the cellular levels to molecular interactions, chemical concentrations, and chemical kinetics. The cell membrane contains docking ports on its surface called receptors that allow the cell to pick up distant chemical signals (hormones, neurotransmitters, prostagladins) sent by other cells through the blood stream and local chemical signals generated by components of the ECM and immune cells. *We will discuss later in this monograph that it is likely that many of these cell receptors also function as antennas for particular frequencies of electromagnetic energy (Haltiwanger, 1998).*

The cell membranes of cancer cells are different from normal cells. Cancer cell membranes have alterations in their lipid/sterol content (Revici, 1961) and in the types of glycoproteins and antigens that they express (Warren et al., 1972; Hakomori, 1990). Cancer cells also exhibit the ability to express their own growth factors and the ability to ignore growth factor inhibition control exerted by the ECM. The extracellular space and the components of the extracellular matrix connect to the cytoskeleton of the cells. The ECM occupies an intermediate space between the intravascular space and the boundary of the cells. The ECM can be considered to function as a pre-kidney, since all substances that have to be eliminated through the bloodstream and kidneys must first pass through the ECM. The ECM is also a transit and storage area for nutrients, water, and waste. The ECM pervades the entire organism and reaches most cells in the body. The CM has anatomic, physical, chemical, and electronic functions. Anatomically, the ECM consists of a recticulum consisting of polymeric protein-sugar complexes bound to water, forming a gel state (Oschman, 2000).

The cytoplasm inside of cells also exists in a gel state. The liquid crystal properties of the molecules in these compartments allow them to undergo cooperative phase transitions in response to changes in temperature, pH, ion concentrations, oxygen concentration, carbon dioxide concentration, ATP concentration, electrical fields, and other physical factors. Cells are organized structures with an internal architecture of cytoskeletal proteins that connect all components of the cell. The enzymes of the cell are attached to the cytoskeletal framework and membranes creating solid-state chemistry (Ho, 1996). Enzymes are not just floating randomly around. Cytoskeletal filaments and tubules form a continuous system that links the cell surface to all organelle structures, including passage through the nuclear membrane to the chromosomes. The cytoskeleton is also attached through cell membrane connectors to liquid crystal protein polymers located in the external ECM and to other cells. The liquid crystal protein polymers of the ECM are mostly composed of collagen, elastin, hylauronic acid, and interweaving glycoproteins such as fibronectin. Fibronectins bind the ECM proteins to each other and to cell membrane integrins. The cell membranes contain proteins called integrins, which creates a continuum linking the internal liquid crystal cytoskeletal proteins to liquid crystal proteins located outside of the cell in the ECM (Oschman, 2000).

When cells become swollen with water (injured cells and cancerous cells), the cell geometry changes which creates different connections, different electron and photon flows, different chemistry, and a different pH. Cancer cells have different cytoskeletal structures, different fat/sterol content in their membranes, different enzymes, and different proteins and cell membrane receptors due to genetic alterations. Some of the proteins of cancer cells are regressive reversions to embryological proteins, which creates different binding and results in loss of connectedness, and different chemistry, especially in energy production. The regressive reversions of cancer cells causes these cells to express different extracellular matrix material creating a more negative charge on the exterior of cancer cells, an alteration in the ionic content inside of cancer cells, and a different interaction with the environment. Physically, the ECM acts as a molecular sieve between the capillaries and the cells (Reichart, 1999).

The concentration of minerals in the ECM, the composition of proteoglycans, the molecular weight of the proteoglycans, the amount of bound water in the ECM, and the pH of the ECM control the filtering aspect of the ECM. The ECM is a transit area for the passage of nutrients from the bloodstream into the cells and for toxins released by the cells that pass through to the bloodstream. It is also a transit area for immune cells that move out of the bloodstream. These immune cells are involved in inflammatory reactions by secreting cytokines and digesting old worn out cells. They may also facilitate healing by carrying and delivering components from other areas of the body to the cell membrane. These migrating immune cells, as well as fixed cells in the ECM, regulate cellular functions by secreting growth factors and cell growth inhibitors (Reichart, 1999). The ECM functions as a storage reservoir for water, nutrients and toxins, and a pH buffering system where the proteins of the ECM buffer acids released by the cells. In healthy conditions, most of the water in the ECM is bound to the interweaving proteoglycans, forming a gel, which creates a physical barrier that limits, directs, and evenly distributes the flow of fluid from the venule end of the capillaries to the cells. When conditions create edema in the ECM, fluid flows more easily from leaky capillaries, but these large flows of fluid are unevenly distributed, which interferes with nutrient delivery, oxygen perfusion, and waste disposal. In edematous conditions, the ECM becomes more hypoxic, more acidic, and electrically more resistant. Bioflavinoids are some of the most effective nutrients in reducing capillary leakage, which helps reduce edema. In a sense, bioflavinoids could be considered to be electrical nutrients because they can help improve the electrical conductivity of the ECM by helping reduce capillary leakage and ECM edema.

Biochemically, the ECM is a metabolically and electrically active space that is involved in regulating cell growth control. Cellular components of the ECM are involved in the local production of growth factors, growth inhibitors, and cytokines that affect the growth and metabolic activity of tissue/organ cells (Reichart, 1999). Immune cells such as leukocytes, lymphocytes, and macrophages that migrate into the ECM are involved in initiating the removal of old and damaged cells and in stimulating the growth of new cells. Fibroblasts and fibrocytes are the main cells that produce the proteins and ground substance of the ECM in soft tissue. The glycocalyx (sugar cell coat) is produced by the cells of parenchymal organs and secreted onto their cell surfaces. The ECM and the glycocalyx work together to regulate information transfer to and from tissue/organ cells by both electrical field fluctuations leading to electro-conformational coupling and soluble signaling molecules.

Electronic functions of the ECM. According to James Oschman, communication systems in living organisms involve two languages: chemical and energetic (Oschman, 2000). Chemical communication in the body takes place mainly through the circulatory system. Energetic communication in the body, according to Western Medical paradigms, takes place almost exclusively in the nervous system. Oschman and Mae Wan Ho (Ho, 1998) have written extensively about an evolutionarily older solid-state electronic communication system that operates both in series and in parallel with the nervous system through the liquid crystal protein polymer connective system continuum. It is through this continuum that information is carried in biological systems via endogenous DC electric fields, their associated magnetic fields and ultra-weak photon emission. This continuum of liquid crystal connections will allow electrons and photons to move in and out of cells. In our opinion, cytoskeletal filaments function as electronic semiconductors and fiberoptic cables, integrating information flow both within the cell and with other cells. This continuum enables an organism to function as a biological hologram. The extracellular connective system is an unrecognized organ that is spread diffusely throughout the body. In medicine, doctors are trained to think of organs as discrete tissues that have particular anatomical locations, but we see the connective tissues as a specialized organ that integrates all parts of the body into a holographic matrix where each organ even each cell is in communication with all other parts. But what about circulating vascular cells and migrating immune cells? They are not attached to connective tissue fibers, so how do they communicate? We believe these cells communicate both by chemical and resonant interactions. We believe that energetic communications in the body take place through hard-wired biologic electronic systems, biologic fiberoptic systems, as well as through resonant interactions. *The electronic functions of the cells and the ECM are involved in healing and tissue regeneration.* Cells are electromagnetic in nature – they generate their own electromagnetic fields and they also harness external electromagnetic energy of the right wavelength and strength to communicate, control, and drive metabolic reactions. The cells of an organism are embedded in a matrix of organized water and most of the body's cells are hardwired into a holographic liquid crystal polymer continuum that connects the cytoskeletal elements of the inside of the cell through cell membrane structures with a semiconducting and fiberoptic liquid crystal polymer connective tissue communication system (Haltiwanger, 1998; Oschman, 2000).

Most of the molecules in the body are electrical dipoles (Beal, 1996). These dipoles electronically *function like transducers* in that they are able to turn *acoustic waves into electrical waves and electrical waves into acoustic waves* (Beal, 1996). The natural properties of biomolecular structures enable cell components and whole cells to oscillate and interact resonantly with other cells (Smith and Best, 1989). According to Smith and Best, the cells of the body and cellular components possess the ability *to function as electrical resonators* (Smith and Best, 1989).

Professor H. Fröhlich has predicted that the fundamental oscillation in cell membranes occurs at frequencies of the order of 100 GHz and that biological systems possess the ability to create and utilize coherent oscillations and respond to external oscillations (Fröhlich, 1988). Lakhovsky predicted that cells possessed this capability in the 1920s (Lakhovsky, 1939).

Because cell membranes are composed of dielectric materials, a cell will behave as a dielectric resonator and will produce an evanescent electromagnetic field in the space around itself (Smith and Best, 1989). "This field does not radiate energy but is capable of interacting with similar systems. Here is the mechanism for the electromagnetic control of biological function" (Smith and Best, 1989). *In our opinion, this means that the applications of certain frequencies by frequency generating devices can enhance or interfere with cellular resonance and cellular metabolic and electrical functions.* Electric fields induce or a cause alignment in dipole movements. A dipole movement is a function of polarization processes and the strength of the electric field. When biological tissue is exposed to an electric field in the right frequency and amplitude windows, a preferential alignment of dipoles becomes established. Since the cell membrane contains many dipole molecules, an electric field will cause preferential alignment of the dipoles. This may be one mechanism that electrical fields alter membrane permeability and membrane functions. Both internally generated and externally applied electromagnetic fields can affect cell functions. The primary external electromagnetic force is the sun, which produces a spectrum of electromagnetic energies. Life evolved utilizing processes that harness the energy of light to produce chemical energy, so in a sense, light is the first nutrient.

Endogenous weak electric fields are naturally present within all living organisms and are apparently involved in pattern-formation and regeneration (Nuccitelli, 1984). Regeneration is a healing process where the body can replace damaged tissues. Some of the most important biophysical factors implicated in tissue repair and regeneration involve the natural electrical properties of the body's tissues and cells (Brighton et al., 1979), such as cell membrane potential and protein semiconduction of electricity. The body utilizes these fundamental bioelectronic features to naturally produce electrical currents that are involved in repair and regeneration (Becker, 1961, 1967, 1970, 1972, 1974, 1990). Robert O. Becker has shown in his research that the flow of endogenous electrical currents in the body is not a secondary process, but in fact is an initiator and control system used by the body to regulate healing in bone and other tissues (Becker, 1970, 1990; Becker and Selden, 1985).

For example, in bone, the proper production and conduction of endogenous electrical currents is required to stimulate primitive precursor cells to differentiate into osteoblasts and chondroblasts (Becker and Selden, 1985; Becker, 1990).

Once the bone-forming osteoblasts are created, they *must maintain a healthy cell membrane electrical potential* and have available certain critical nutrients in order to form the polysaccharide and collagen components of osteoid. Endogenous bone electrical currents created through piezoelectricity (Fukada, 1957, 1984) are also required for deposition of calcium crystals (Becker et al., 1964). *When the biophysical electrical properties of the tissues are considered, it makes sense to develop therapeutic strategies that support the body's biophysical electrical processes to potentiate the healing of injured, diseased, and cancerous tissues.*

The ECM-glycocalyx-membrane interface. Cell membranes are composed of phospholipids, sterols, and embedded or attached proteins. The composition of the cell membrane directly affects cell *membrane functions* which include membrane permeability, cell signaling, and cell capacitance. Glycoproteins secreted from the cell interior and cellular components of the ECM create the glycocalyx covering of cells. Some of these glycoproteins are components of cell membrane receptors, making them important in signaling processes such as activation by growth factors. These glycoproteins characteristically have a negative electrical charge. Cancer cells, however, have excessively high concentrations of negatively-charged molecules on their exterior surface, which act as electric shields (Cure, 1991, 1995). Cell membrane glycoproteins act as molecular chemical receptors and electromagnetic or electric field antennas (Adey, 1988). If Adey is correct, then cells function both as chemical and *electrical receivers and transmitters. Signaling mechanisms may be either chemically or resonantly mediated.* Chemical communication is mediated by chemical soluble signals that travel through the bloodstream and then through the ECM from distant locations or chemicals that are locally produced in the ECM. These soluble signaling molecules may be produced in distant sites by endocrine cells or are secreted by cells embedded within the ECM or cells that migrate into the ECM such as macrophages, T-cells, and B-cells.

When these soluble signaling molecules are presented to the organ cells, they can either activate or inhibit cellular metabolic reactions by activating cell membrane or cytoplasmic glycoprotein receptors (Reichart, 1999). Chemical signal activation of cell receptors will cause the receptor's molecular structure to shift from an inactive to an activated conformational state. This is a phase transition. When a receptor is activated, it will bind to and activate other membrane bound proteins or intracellular proteins/enzymes. The outcome of receptor activation may increase the transport of certain molecules or mineral ions from one side of the cell membrane to the other side, increase or inhibit the activity of enzymes involved in metabolic synthesis or degradation, activate genes to produce certain proteins, turn off gene production of other proteins, or cause cytoskeletal proteins to change the shape or motility of the cell. When the receptor protein switches back to its inactive conformation, it will detach from the effector proteins/enzymes and the signal will cease (Van Winkle, 1995). Cell receptors can also be activated by electric fields (vibrational resonance) that have particular frequencies and amplitudes through a process known as *electro-conformational coupling* (Tsong, 1989). Electrical oscillations of the right frequency and amplitude can alter the electrical charge distribution in cell receptors, causing the cell receptors to undergo conformational changes just as if the receptor were activated by a chemical signal. Ross Adey has extensively described in his publications that the application of weak electromagnetic fields of certain windows of frequency and intensity act as first messengers by activating glycoprotein receptors in the cell membrane (Adey, 1993). This electrical property of cell receptor-membrane complexes would allow cells to scan incoming frequencies and tune their circuitry to allow them to resonate at particular frequencies (Charman, 1996).

Adey and other researchers have reported that one effect of the application of weak electromagnetic fields is the release of calcium ions inside of the cell (Adey, 1993). Adey has also documented that cells respond constructively to a wide range of frequencies, including frequencies in the extremely low frequency (ELF) range of 1-10 Hz, which is a range of frequencies known as the Schumann resonance frequencies that are naturally produced in the atmosphere (Adey, 1993). Adey has also reported that certain frequency bands between 15-60 Hz have been found to promote cancers. Frequencies in this range have been found to alter cell protein synthesis, mRNA functions, immune responses, and intercellular communication (Adey, 1992). The ECM also contains nerve fibers connected through the autonomic nervous system back to the brain, which then regulates hormone homeostasis by feedback control through the hypothalamic pituitary axis.

Resonance Communication Mechanisms

The ground substance of the ECM contains an electrical field that will fluctuate in response to the composition of proteoglycans, especially the degree of negative charge, which is dependent on the concentration of sialic acid residues and the ion/mineral content of the ECM. The fluctuations/oscillations of the electric field of the ECM, when strong enough, can lead to local depolarization of portions of the cell membrane and changes in membrane permeability. The oscillation of the electrical potential can affect, through resonance (electrochemical coupling), the conformational structures of cell membrane receptors. The receptors can switch back and forth between conformations, which will lead to turning on the activity of membrane-embedded enzymes and opening and closing ion channels. Electrical field fluctuations that occur in the ECM and these field fluctuations are involved in cell signaling mechanisms. A number of researchers such as Becker and Adey believe that natural weak endogenous electric fields actually control the chemical process of cell membrane signaling. *This means that measures that enhance or disturb the production of these natural electric fields can impact cell-signaling processes.* In the future, electrical medicine will advance to the point where you can dial up and administer frequencies that will act like pharmacological agents. When this occurs, the phrase 'beam me up Scottie' may take on a whole new meaning.

The natural oscillating electrical potential of the ECM can be adversely affected or constructively supported by exposure to external electromagnetic fields. Adverse electromagnetic field exposure can be initiated by exposure to high power tension lines, transformers, and electronic equipment such as cell phones. Constructive support includes use of *certain nutrients* and devices like infrared emitters, phototherapy equipment, multiwave oscillators, and microcurrent equipment that emit electromagnetic fields and electrical currents in physiological ranges. Acoustical (sound) waves of the right frequency can also affect cell-signaling and cellular metabolic processes.

The Bioelectrical Control System

The body uses electricity (biocurrents) as part of the body's mechanism for controlling growth and repair (Borgens et al., 1989). Some of these biocurrents travel through hydrated liquid crystal semiconducting protein-proteoglycan (collagen-hyaluronic acid) complexes of the ECM. Key elements that support this physiologic function include proper hydration and normal protein configurations, which allow for the water to be structured in concentric nanometer thick layers (Ling, 2001). The production of normal ECM components and proper ion concentrations are also important. Healthy production of collagen and hyaluronic acid in the ECM is, in turn, dependent upon the interactions of internal cellular machinery that produces proteins and sugars, especially proper reading of the genetic code, availability of construction material like amino acids such as lysine and proline that are needed for collagen production, intracellular availability of cofactors of protein and sugar producing enzymes such as zinc, magnesium, trace minerals, vitamin C, bioflavinoids, and B-complex vitamins, and the availability of endogenously produced and ingested precursor molecules such as glucosamine, mannose, galactose, etc. Biocurrents in the ECM pass through the cell membrane into the cell while electrons produced in the cell also pass out through the cell membrane.

Dr. Merrill Garnett has spent four decades studying the role of charge transfer and electrical current flow in the cell (Garnett, 1998). Dr. Garnett believes that biological liquid crystal molecules and structures such as hyaluronic acid, prothrombin, DNA, cytoskeletal proteins, and cell membranes are involved in maintaining both an inward and outward current. The inward current flows from the cell membrane to cell structures like mitochondria and DNA and the outward current flows back along liquid crystal semiconducting cytoskeletal proteins back through the cell membrane to the ECM. Dr. Garnett has reported that all cancer cells have abnormal electron transfer systems and that normal cell development involves normal energy flows (Garnett, 1998). Dr. Garnett believes that electrical charges stored in the cell membrane (capacitance) and electrical charges of oxygen free radicals are normally transferred to DNA and are involved in DNA activation and the creation of an electrical field around DNA. DNA is very effective in transferring large amounts of electrical charge along its long axis (Garnett, 1998). In fact, new research shows that DNA molecules may be good molecular semiconductors (Li and Yan, 2001). Dr. Garnett believes that an electrical pathway from the cell membrane fats to DNA is a natural pathway, related to development in cells that use aerobic mechanisms of ATP production (Garnett, 1998).

As a corollary, this natural electrical pathway is *transiently disrupted* in healthy cells while they are involved in wound healing and permanently disrupted in cancer cells that rely on anaerobic glycolysis for energy production. He believes that cells that are transformed into cancer cells have highly altered energy metabolism that includes increased reliance on glycolysis and a shift to the use of glutamine in the TCA cycle (Garnett, 1998). Cancer cells and normal cells that are growing in hypoxic areas use anaerobic energy production pathways that are regressions to earlier stages of embryonic development, but unlike normal cells that reverse back to aerobic metabolism, cancer cells remain permanently locked into the anaerobic method of energy production. He has theorized that an alternating current oscillating circuit exists inside of cells between the cell membrane and the DNA that is conducted over electronic protein polymers inside of the cell. This circuit is activated during differentiation to trigger the expression of genes (Garnett et al., 2002). *If Garnett is correct, then it means that cells use their electrical properties to control gene expression.* Garnett has hypothesized that the part of the DNA coiled around protein structures called nucleosomes may exhibit electronic inductance. "As a coil, it has electronic inductance, and since we have a series of coils, we have a series inductance circuit. DNA current passes initially through the helix in a state where it can discharge its field energy. Hence we have a pulse within the DNA interacting with other biomolecules like the membrane. The pulse can go in and come out, and the DNA is not imperiled" (Garnett, 2000). He has subsequently developed, after thousands of attempts, a water-soluble and fat-soluble liquid crystal polymer compound composed of palladium and lipoic acid (Poly MVA) that is able to enter the cell and reestablish the electrical connection between the cell membrane and DNA. Garnett's research shows that liquid crystal polymers like prothrombin, hyaluronic acid, and palladium-lipoic acid complex (Poly MVA) normally produces fern structures. *In our opinion, these types of structures are molecular antennas and electrical conductors.* This new nontoxic drug acts as an electrical shunt that causes cells that utilize anaerobic glycolysis to undergo membrane rupture and die while leaving aerobic cells that utilize efficient oxygen-dependent electron transfer undamaged (Garnett, 1998; Garnett and Remo, 2001). Aerobic cells are protected from this electrocution because their functional mitochondria normally engage in electron transport ending with oxygen as the final electron acceptor (Garnett and Remo, 2001).

Electrical Properties of the ECM

The proteoglycans that compose the ground substance of the ECM are negatively-charged. The number and type of sialic acid residues that cap the glycoproteins of the cell coat also determine the degree of negative charge of the cell surface. The negative charges of the ECM-glycocalyx interface help determine water balance, ion balance, and osmotic balance both in the ground substance of the ECM and inside of the cells. The ECM proteoglycans exist in fern shapes that allow electric charges to flow and disorganized shapes that impair transit through the ECM of electrical currents and nutrients. These disorganized shapes occur when tissue inflammation is present and toxins are present in the ECM. These factors create areas of high electrical resistance. Tissues of the body that are injured have a higher electrical resistance than the surrounding tissue. The cell membranes of these tissues become less permeable to the flow of ions and more electrically-insulated. This results in the endogenous bioelectric currents avoiding these areas of high resistance (Wing, 1989). The reduction in electrical flow through an injured area is one factor that interferes with healing. Increasing the electrical resistance of a tissue will impede the flow of healing biocurrents

(Becker, 1985). Decreasing the electrical flow through an injured area also results in a decrease of the membrane capacitance of the cells in that area. Conversely, improving the electrical conductance of the ECM will improve healing and improve cell membrane charge. Correction of tissue inflammation and ECM toxicity can improve the electrical functions of the ECM. Therefore, the composition and degree of toxicity of the ECM-glycocalyx interface will affect the electrical field and the flow of biocurrents in the ECM. The electrical field and biocurrent conduction in the ECM in turn will affect cell membrane capacitance, permeability of the cell membrane, signaling mechanisms of the cell membrane, intracellular mineral concentrations, nutrient flow into the cell, and waste disposal (Wing, 1989; Oschman, 2000).

The ECM can be cleared of toxins by a variety of measures. Detoxification strategies could include the use of antioxidants and the support of antioxidant pathways, oral enzymes, homeopathic and herbal preparations, chelation (IV and oral), infrasonic devices, multiwave oscillators, microcurrent devices, and phototherapy devices (lasers and LEDS). Some clinicians use live blood microscopy to see if their therapies are increasing the entry of wastes into the bloodstream. If a live blood slide shows a marked increase in wastes after a treatment compared to a slide obtained before treatment, then the clinician can tell that his or her treatment is cleaning the walls of blood vessels and removing toxins from the extracellular space. The body's biocurrents and the electrical field of the ECM controls cell differentiation and the metabolic activity of mature cells. Mesenchymal cells will differentiate under the influence of electrical fields: fibroblasts to fibrocytes, myoblasts to myocytes, chondroblasts to chondrocytes, and osteoblasts to osteocytes (Becker, 1985). The bioelectric control system's contribution to cell differentiation and cell growth can be assisted by the use of certain types of waters that enhance the liquid crystal properties of ECM polymers, promoting cell production of ECM proteins and proteoglycans, providing exogenous growth factor control and mediators of inflammation, promoting internal production of growth factors, and inflammatory mediator by ECM cells and other factors.

Pathology of the ECM

The ECM can be a storage site for nutrients or it can be a dumping ground for toxins, which can disrupt the metabolic and electrical functions of the ECM. Deposition of pathological deposits of proteins and toxins can lead to degenerative processes (e.g., amyloid can lead to Alzheimer's and immune complex deposition can lead to autoimmune inflammation). Inflammatory processes can lead to the deposition of crystals, calcium, cholesterol, and edema. The ECM is a buffering system for acids excreted by the cells. Impairment in the ability to excrete these acids or over-production of acids by metabolic dysregulation will first lead to acidification of the ECM. Chronic acidification of the ECM will eventually lead to increased acidification of the intracellular compartment, which can create impairment of cellular metabolic processes, especially aerobic energy production. Eventually, disruption of cellular organelle functions and structures will occur. Excessive acidification of the ECM will eventually lead to saturation of the buffering capacity of ECM proteins. This will result in mobilization of calcium, magnesium, and heavy metals from the skeleton. When calcium, magnesium, and other minerals are chronically mobilized from the bone for use as mineral buffers, these minerals will be lost through the kidneys and will create total body depletion of these minerals. Excessive and prolonged acidic conditions will result in increased mineral mobilization from the skeleton. Such a condition will first create osteopenia and, in the long run, will eventually progress to osteoporosis and compression fractures. Increased mobilization of heavy metals will lead to metabolic stress on the kidneys as these organs attempt to excrete these metals by use of glutathione detoxification. If the glutathione system becomes depleted due to excessive toxic burden, these heavy metals will accumulate in the kidneys. Heavy metal accumulation in the kidneys may account for 1/6 of the cases of hypertension in middle-aged people. This mechanism is one reason that the incidence of hypertension rises in post-menopausal women. *In our experience, supporting kidney glutathione detoxification can reduce hypertension in some individuals.*

This section contains information about:

1. The different intracellular mineral concentrations in tumors
2. pH alterations in tumors
3. How to alter intracellular pH in cancers
4. Tumor hypoxic regions
5. Tumor cell coats and the role of hCG and sialic acid
6. The low transmembrane potential of cancer cells
7. How to increase low transmembrane potential in cancer cells
8. How to increase intracellular mineral concentrations of potassium, magnesium, and calcium when low mineral conditions exist in malignant tissues
9. The role of Nieper minerals transporters
10. And why the number 42 is the universal answer to all questions

Mineral and water abnormalities in cancerous and injured tissues: sodium, potassium, magnesium and calcium and their effect on cell membrane potential. The cell membrane is a dividing structure that maintains biochemically-distinct compartments between the inside (intracellular) and outside (extracellular) spaces (Marieb 1998). The lipid structure of a cell membrane makes it relatively impermeable to the passage of charged molecules. Therefore, charged molecules must cross through ion channels. Ion channels are transmembrane protein molecules that contain aqueous pores connecting the inside of the cell to the extracellular space. These channels can open and shut in response to a variety of signals. The passage of charged molecules through ion channels in the cell membrane endows the membrane with an electrical conductive property allowing for inward and outward current flows (Aidley and Stanfield, 1996). This is one factor that establishes electric circuits in biological tissues. In order to maintain balance in intracellular fluid and electrolytes, water, sodium, and potassium are in constant motion between the intracellular and extracellular compartments (Edwards 1998). Extracellular fluids and intracellular fluids contain different concentrations of minerals. These minerals carry positive charges and are called cations. In order to maintain electric neutrality negatively-charged molecules called anions must match these cations in concentration. Sodium is the main cation of ECF whereas potassium is the major cation of ICF. Chloride and bicarbonate are the main anions of ECF, while proteins and organic phosphates are the main anions of ICF. Uncharged molecules such as glucose or urea are also present in both compartments (Edwards, 1998). The passage of electrically-charged ions through a membrane will create a flow of electric currents through the membrane. These ions in turn will affect the metabolism of the cell and the potential of the cell membrane. So it would be expected that all living cells of the body would naturally have a weak electric current flowing through them. In fact, there are bioelectrical circuits continually circulating throughout the body (Stanish, 1985). Overall mineral, water, and membrane changes in cancerous tissues play important roles in changing the cellular geometry, metabolic biochemistry, and electrical properties of cancer cells. Keith Brewer has reported that intracellular calcium and magnesium concentrations are lower in cancer cells due to impaired membrane transport (Brewer, 1985). According to Brewer, the transport of substances across the cell membrane is controlled by the electrical properties of the chemical bonds on and in the membrane, the electrical gradient across the membrane, and the electrical attractions between positively-charged cations and polar molecules with positive and negative regions (Brewer and Passwater, 1976). F.W. Cope in his writings has described a characteristic pattern of electrolyte and fluid abnormalities that occur in any tissue that is damaged. He calls this pattern the 'tissue damage syndrome.' When cells are injured from any cause, cells will lose potassium and accumulate sodium and water (Cope, 1978). According to Cope, the proteins of a healthy cell exist in normal electronic configurational state where a significant proportion of cell water is structured or bound in concentric rings around the protein molecules. In addition, when the proteins are in their healthy configuration, the negatively-charged sites on the protein matrix will have a greater preference for association with potassium rather than with sodium (Cope, 1978). If Cope is correct, this may be one of the factors that accounts for the finding that healthy cells have high cell potassium and low cell sodium concentrations. A number of proteins are present within the cell and in the ECM. Other proteins lie on the inner and outer surface of cell membranes and some are embedded within the cell membrane. These proteins consist of linear chains of amino acid residues with attached carbohydrate and or lipid molecules. The electro attractive and repulsive forces between these components and the external or internal saltwater environment cause these proteins to fold into three-dimensional shapes called conformational states. Protein function is dependent on these conformational states. The cell membrane and its associated membrane proteins are dynamically active with the associated proteins undergoing continuous changes in state. In proteins that are enzymes, the conformational state determines whether or not the enzyme will expose its ligand binding sites.

But if the membrane protein is an ion channel, the conformational structure will determine whether the channel is open or closed. When the channel is open, it is able to pass ions such as potassium, sodium, chloride, and calcium across the cell membrane (Hille, 1992). The cell membrane is impermeable to ions unless its protein-based ion channels are open. Normally, the cell membrane establishes different concentrations of charged ions on either side of the membrane. This cell membrane property creates an electrical potential across the membrane. The ability of the cell proteins to stay in their normal configurational state is dependent on the cell being free from chemical, physical, or hypoxic damage. When physical, chemical, or hypoxic damage occurs to a cell, many cell proteins will change to an abnormal damaged configurational state. In that state "the cell proteins lose their preference for association with potassium rather than sodium, and lose much of their ability to structure water" (Cope, 1978).

When these protein changes occur, potassium leaves the cell and is replaced by sodium. In addition, the water content and the percentage of unbound water within the cell increases (the cell swells) (Ling and Ochsenfeld, 1976). Proteins can also be induced to resume their normal configuration by measures that increase the intracellular concentration of potassium, magnesium, and ATP. This will result in cell water becoming more structured and will cause the cell to release unstructured cell water and sodium (Cope, 1978). *Note: magnesium is involved in maintaining the intracellular concentration of potassium.* The structuring of water around intracellular proteins will also affect the configurational state, liquid crystal, and electrical properties of these proteins. Structured or bound water has less freedom of movement than unbound water. Nuclear magnetic resonance (NMR) can be used to measure the amount of water that is structured in normal and cancerous cells. Hazelwood and his colleagues showed in a 1974 NMR study that malignant tissues have significantly increased amounts of unbound water compared to normal tissues (Hazelwood, 1984).

The changes in the degree that water is structured in a cell or in the ECM will affect the configurations and liquid crystal properties of proteins, cell membranes, organelle membranes, and DNA. *Healthy tissues have more structured water than unhealthy tissues. Clinicians who recognize this fact have found that certain types of music, toning, chanting, tuning forks, singing bowls, magnetic waters, certain types of frequency generators, phototherapy treatments, and homeopathic preparations can improve water structuring in the tissues and health when they are correctly utilized.* In cancer, a number of features such as changes in the mineral concentrations inside of the cell, the degree that water is structured inside of the cell, and an excess of negative electrical charges on the exterior surface of the cell cause the cell membrane potential of cancerous cells to be less than normal (Cone, 1970). Cancerous tissues and less-differentiated regenerating tissues are more electronegative than normal cells and normal tissues (Ambrose et al., 1969; Schaubel et al., 1970; Becker, 1985).

Cone reported in 1975 that the electrical potential of cancer cell membranes was significantly less than the membrane electrical potential of healthy cells. Basically, the lower membrane potential of cancer cells is associated with higher intracellular sodium concentrations and lower intracellular potassium concentrations (Cone, 1975). Cone found that healthy cells have higher intracellular potassium, lower intracellular sodium, and higher electrical cell membrane potential, while cancer cells have higher sodium, lower potassium, and lower membrane electrical potential. As a result of increased intracellular sodium, cancer cells will retain more water, causing them to be more spherical and have different geometry than normal cells. When cells become swollen with too much water, normal cell signaling mechanisms are disrupted, aerobic cellular metabolism of sugars is inhibited, and ATP production falls. Intracellular sodium has a mitotic regulating effect. Clarence D. Cone, Jr. has postulated that an unfavorable intracellular sodium-potassium ratio with excessive intracellular sodium and low intracellular potassium could affect the transmembrane potential of malignant cells (Cone, 1975) and predispose a cell to malignant mitogenesis (Regelson, 1980). Tumor cell differentiation, tumor hypoxia, and low cellular pH can affect gene expression, genetic stability, genetic repair, protein structures, protein activity, intracellular mineral concentrations, and types of metabolic pathways used for energy production. Cancers often exhibit increasingly malignant behavior during their growth. Why? One reason is that cancerous tumors are composed of cell populations that range from highly-aggressive undifferentiated cells to well-differentiated cells. Some cancers are almost completely composed of undifferentiated cells that are biochemically similar to embryonic cells because of increased expression of embryonic genes. Highly-undifferentiated tumors typically produce gene products such as proteins like alpha-fetoprotein (AFP) and carcinoembryonic antigen (CEA), enzymes and hormones such as human chorionic gonadotropin (hCG) that are characteristic of embryonic tissues. On the other hand, tumors with well-differentiated cells will produce gene products more closely resembling normal adult tissues. In general, tumors with highly-undifferentiated cells are more invasive than tumors composed of well-differentiated cells or tumors with mixed cell populations.

Increased malignant behavior during tumor growth is also affected by the microenvironment of tumors, which is characterized by fluctuating areas of both acute and chronic hypoxia, low pH, and nutrient deprivation (Moulder et al., 1987; Rockwell, 1992). The severity of hypoxia and acidosis in tumors can affect tumor cell invasiveness, metastasis, the risk of recurrence and resistance to chemotherapy and radiation therapy (Teicher, 1994; Rofstad, 2000). Tumors exist in a dynamic Darwinian state of survival of the fittest. Tumors continually secrete growth factors that initiate the formation of new blood vessels, yet many tumors grow so rapidly that they out-grow their blood supply so that large tumors will have areas that are poorly oxygenated (hypoxic) and other areas that are well-oxygenated (Vaupel et al., 1991). Hypoxic and well-oxygenated areas will actually fluctuate coming and going as blood vessels form and then regress (Holash et al., 1999). Tumors with areas of mixed oxygenation will often contain heterogeneous groups of cells that exhibit biochemical diversity. The same tumor will have some cells that are utilizing different metabolic reactions to create energy than other groups of cells in the same tumor. This is one reason why different cell populations in the same tumor will respond differently to treatment measures. Some cells will be killed by a particular treatment while other cells will survive and, in a sense, be selected for further growth (Gray et al., 1953; Graeber et al., 1996). Fluctuating oxygen levels will result in fluctuations in the types of genes that are activated, types of proteins that are produced, and the types of metabolic reactions that occur (Dang et al., 1997).

Fluctuations in the types of metabolic reactions used to create energy will result in variations in lactic acid production, acid excretion, and acid accumulation both within the cells and in within the ECM. In vitro studies have shown that tumor cell surface adhesion molecules are down-regulated upon exposure to hypoxia conditions (Hasan et al., 1998). This means that hypoxia can result in decreased cell adhesion of tumor cells to the ECM. Loss of contact with the ECM permits tumor cells to spread to more distant locations and reduces the ability of the ECM to exert growth inhibition. Some researchers have focused on the finding that the hypoxic and acidic microenvironment of tumors will create further genetic instability and mutations (Reynolds et al., 1996). Hypoxia and acidic tumor microenvironments will cause certain genes to become activated and expressed and other genes to be inactivated so that the metabolic reactions of tumor cells will be altered. These conditions can also create DNA damage and impair DNA repair mechanisms (Yuan et al., 1998, 2000). Low intracellular pH can alter the conformational structure and function of cellular proteins, including DNA polymerases (Eckert and Kunkel, 1993). One common characteristic of many tumors is the reduced activity of a special protein called p53 that is involved in triggering cell death. Hypoxic conditions will favor selection of tumor cells with reduced apoptotic potential (Graeber et al., 1999). Tumor cells that are hypoxic lack sufficient oxygen to activate their aerobic metabolic pathways. These cells will typically begin to rely on anaerobic metabolism to supply their energy needs (Rossi-Fanelli et al., 1991). Tumor cells in hypoxic conditions will convert most of their pyruvate to lactate instead of to acetyl Coenzyme A (Warburg, 1956). This type of energy production is very inefficient, so tumors require much larger amounts of sugar in order to maintain their energy production. Tumor cells, in a sense, become sugar junkies.

Tumor cells express several adaptations in order to sustain their sugar addiction and metabolic strategies to address this issue. Tumor cells will express larger amounts of glucose receptors/transporters on their cell surface in order to increase their sugar uptake (Van Winkle, 1999). In fact hypoxia stimulates the transcription of numerous genes including genes that code for enzymes of the glycolytic pathway and cell membrane glucose transport proteins GLUT-1 and GLUT-3 (Semenza, 2002). The administration of cesium salts has been reported to limit tumor cell uptake of glucose, which starves the cancer cell and reduces its ability to make energy by fermentation. Tumor cells will increase the activity of an intracellular enzyme called glucokinase. An extract of avocado called mannoheptulose has been found to inhibit glucose entry into tumor cells and reduce the activity of glucokinase – an enzyme that sequesters sugar inside of the cell (Board et al., 1995). Some tumor cells express glycoproteins that promote protein breakdown (Stipanuk, 2000). The secretion of cytokines, especially tumor necrosis factor, increases in cancer. Some of these cytokines increase the breakdown of tissue proteins (Bender, 2002). The amino acids released by protein breakdown can be used in gluconeogenesis. Tumor necrosis factor not only promotes protein breakdown, but it also increases gluconeogenesis (Bender, 2002). Many tumor cells will produce lactate when they metabolize glucose anaerobically. The lactate is exported from the tumor cells and is utilized by the liver in gluconeogenesis (Bender, 2002).

Overall gluconeogenesis is stimulated when cancer is present. Gluconeogenesis requires a great deal of energy and excessive gluconeogenesis is thought to be a significant factor that contributes to cancer cachexia (Gold, 1968). Dr. Joseph Gold recognized in the 1960s that metabolic strategies that inhibited the enzyme phosphoenol pyruvate carboxykinase (PEP-CK) would reduce gluconeogenesis and decrease the severity of cachexia (Gold, 1968). Dr. Gold, after testing a series of compounds, found that hydrazine sulfate could effectively reduce excessive gluconeogenesis in cancer (Gold, 1974, 1981).

Tumor acidification versus tumor alkalization. One of the characteristic features of cancers is that cancerous cells rapidly divide and proliferate. In general, growing cancers have many cells that are undergoing mitosis. According to Keith Brewer, normal and malignant cells undergo mitosis between a pH range of 6.5 – 7.5 and the mitosis rate slows as the intracellular pH approaches the extremes of this range. If a cell can be forced into a pH outside of this range, cell division ceases (Brewer, 1985). Recognition of this fact serves as the basis for therapies that increase or decrease the pH of tumor cells. When it was first discovered that tumors utilize anaerobic metabolism of glucose, it was thought that providing more oxygen would convert tumors back to aerobic metabolism (Warburg, 1930). Unfortunately, tumors still exhibit high levels of glycolysis even under aerobic conditions

(Weinhouse, 1976). Because glycolytic metabolism predominates in tumors some lactic acid accumulation and intracellular acidification may occur in tumors under hypoxic conditions although most of the lactic acid and hydrogen ions are exported into the ECM, leading to acidification of the ECM (Ojugo et al., 1999). The extracellular pH around tumor tissues is usually more acidic than the extracellular pH of normal tissues. Extracellular pH levels as low as 7.09 have been measured in some human tumors (Van der Zee et al., 1989). It is thought that both lactate and hydrogen protons are exported from tumor cells into the extracellular space as a way of limiting intracellular acidity (Ojugo et al., 1999). Tumor cells are so efficient in sequestering and exporting acids that they are often able to maintain their cytoplasmic pH nearly equal to that of normal cells, which is about 7.0 - 7.3 (Newell et al., 1993; Stubbs at al., 1994). Intracellular cytoplasmic pH is maintained in tumor cells by sequestration of acids in cytoplasmic vesicles and cell membrane mechanisms that include a sodium hydrogen ion exchanger, lactate transport out of tumor cells, and chloride and bicarbonate exchange (Webb et al., 1999). Sodium movement into the cells enables the membrane exchange system to pump hydrogen ions out of the cell (Mahnensmith and Aronson, 1985). The net result of activating the sodium- hydrogen ion exchanger is that *sodium accumulates inside of tumor cells.* Intracellular concentrations of sodium are typically higher in malignant cells than in normal cells (Cone, 1975; Cope, 1978; Seeger and Wolz, 1990; Cure, 1991, 1995). Although tumor cells are relatively-efficient in exporting acid (hydrogen protons) into the ECM and sequestering acids in cytoplasmic vesicles, we believe the buildup of intracellular acids in cytoplasmic vesicles may still possibly interfere with mitochondrial production of ATP by disrupting the hydrogen ion gradient across the mitochondrial membrane. This would create a positive feedback loop where anaerobic glycolysis creates an intracellular acidic condition that further interferes with oxygen-mediated electron transport in the mitochondria. Therefore, in order to maintain energy, anaerobic glycolysis would be continued.

Tumor acidification. When agents are used to block the movement of lactate and hydrogen protons from tumor cells, the effects of therapies that increase cellular acidification are enhanced. Blockage of the export of lactic acid will result in a significant reduction in intracellular pH.

Augmentation of tumor acidification by increasing lactic acid production and blocking tumor cell lactate excretion. The bioflavinoid quercitin has been found to inhibit the synthesis of heat shock proteins in tumors and to block the export of lactate from tumors creating lethal levels of intracellular acidity (Kim et al., 1984). The use of quercitin as a cancer treatment has been the subject of several patents. Unfortunately, this treatment is generally effective only in the hypoxic portion of tumors and is generally ineffective in tumors and areas of tumors that are not hypoxic. Use of quercitin is most effective when hyperthermic treatments are used concurrently. The creation of a hyperglycemic condition can contribute to further intracellular acidification. A number of researchers have reported regarding the use of oral and IV glucose as a way to increase tumor acidity (Volk et al., 1993; Leeper et al., 1998). Research studies have shown that extracellular acidification of tumors will enhance the effect of hyperthermia (Gerweck, 1977; Wike-Hooley, 1984; van de Merwe et al., 1993) and inhibit the development of thermotolerance in cultured tumor cells (Goldin and Leeper, 1981). Manfred von Ardenne of Germany was one of the pioneers who, back in the 1960s, began developing a treatment of cancer utilizing IV glucose to create increased levels of tumor acidity. He would then use hyperthermia to kill cancer cells that were already compromised by excessive acidity (von Ardenne, 1994). Cancer researchers are studying the use of both intracellular and extracellular acidification of tumors to enhance the cytotoxic effects of chemotherapeutic agents (Atema et al., 1993; Skarsgard et al., 1995; Kuin et al., 1999).

Tumor alkalization. Cesium is a naturally-occurring alkaline element that was promoted for use in cancer by a scientist named Keith Brewer, since cesium is preferentially taken up by tumor cells (Brewer, 1985). Use of Cesium is thought to reduce the cellular uptake of glucose by cancer cells, leading to starvation of the cell. Cesium also was reported by Brewer to raise the cell pH of cancer cells up to a range of 8.0. Brewer thought that raising the pH of cancer cells this high would kill cancer cells. The use of cesium in cancer has met with mixed results (Sartori, 1984). *We caution anyone who might be tempted to use this treatment to read extensively about cesium before administering this compound.* The pH of the intracellular and extracellular compartments will also affect the intracellular potassium concentration.

Acidic and alkaline conditions. Cellular uptake of potassium is postulated to be regulated by a membrane-associated energy and magnesium-dependent sodium/potassium pump. Although Dr. Gilbert Ling has a completely different opinion of the mechanisms that cells use to regulate intracellular potassium concentrations (Ling, 2001), he basically believes that the membrane pump theory is wrong. He has extensively published information on his association-induction (AI) hypothesis, which includes the idea that ATP bonding to intracellular proteins mediates selective and preferential absorption of potassium over sodium (Ling, 2001). We find Dr. Ling's work to be highly technical, but very informative. Movement of potassium out of the cell interior is regulated by acidity of the cell interior, the permeability of the cell membrane, and chemical and electrical gradients to the potassium ions. Accumulation of positively-charged hydrogen cations inside of the cells through either respiratory or metabolic acidosis will promote a shift of potassium out of the cells, leading to higher than normal levels of potassium in the bloodstream (hyperkalaemia), lower than normal potassium intracellularly, and increased potassium loss through the kidneys. When intracellular acidity develops from alterations in intracellular metabolism, such as occurs in anaerobic metabolism, excessive amounts of hydrogen ions are created inside of the cell. Cancer cells attempt to reduce cytoplasmic hydrogen cation concentrations by exporting the hydrogen cations into the EC space and by compartmentalizing the hydrogen cations in cytoplasmic storage vesicles (Webb et al., 1999).

The accumulation of excess in positive charge will cause cancer cells to export both hydrogen ions and potassium in order to maintain electrical neutrality. This appears to me to be one more way that cancer cells lose potassium. When cancer cells export hydrogen ions, the ECF space becomes more acidic (lower pH). The amount of acids produced by cancer cells may even be severe enough to overwhelm the body's homeostatic pH regulatory mechanisms. Cancer cells as a group are very efficient in exporting and compartmentalizing hydrogen cations. Some cancer cells are so efficient that they actually become more alkaline than normal cells, but other cancer cells that are not able to completely reduce the concentration of positively charged hydrogen ions in their cytoplasm will have a pH that is typically lower than nonmalignant cells. The studies we found on cancer cell pH showed that there was diversity in intracellular pH levels. In general, cancer cells in hypoxic areas will have to deal with larger amounts of acid. The cell cytoplasm of malignant cells may or may not be acidic depending on how efficient tumor cells are in sequestering and exporting acids. But the ECM around tumor cells is acidic. By definition, acidic tissues are electron-deficient. So a tumor may have areas that have a relative state of electron deficiency. *This condition of electron deficiency may help explain why measures that increase electron availably, like magnetized waters, lemon juice, negative ion generators, standing by waterfalls, standing by the ocean surf, use of electron rich antioxidants, consumption of electron dense foods (fresh vegetables and vegetable juices and essential fatty acids like fresh flax oil) help some people with chronic degenerative conditions and cancers get better. Note: many chronic degenerative conditions are associated with tissue acidity.* Awareness of such findings gives credence to nutritional approaches to cancer, such as the dietary program advocated by Max B. Gerson. Dr. Gerson, during his medical career, advocated low sodium intake and high potassium supplementation through use of raw vegetable juices and potassium supplementation (Cope, 1978; Ling, 1983). Tumor cell coats contain human chorionic gonadotropin and sialic acid as well as negatively-charged residues of RNA, which give tumor cells a strong negative charge on their cell surface All cells have cell surface glycoproteins. As cells specialize, they develop unique sets of cell surface glycoproteins that allow cells of the same type to recognize, communicate, and adhere to each other (Reichart, 1999). These cell surface glycoproteins contain varying concentrations of sialic acid, which is one of the primary molecules responsible for conferring a negative charge to the cell surface of all cells (Cure, 1995; Acevedo et al., 1998). The chemical characteristics of hCG make it a sialoglycoprotein (Acevedo, 2002). Human chorionic gonadotropin (hCG) is a hormone usually associated with pregnancy, however hCG or subunits of hCG can be found on the surface of all cancer cells (Acevedo et al., 1998; Acevedo, 2002). Dr. Acevedo has proposed that the presence of hCG on the surface of cancer cells is a universal marker for cancer (Acevedo et al., 1995; Acevedo, 2002). According to Dr. Acevedo, malignant transformation will cause the genes that code for hCG to become activated, causing cancer cells to begin producing this hormone (Acevedo, 2002). When cancer cells secrete this hormone, it collects on the cell surface. Since hCG contains large amounts of sialic acid, this results in cancer cells having a stronger cell surface negative charge than normal cells (Acevedo et al., 1998).

Cure, in his papers, presents data that cancer cells are also coated by negatively-charged residues of RNA, which is another contributing factor to the strong cell surface negative charge of cancer cells (Cure, 1991, 1995). Cure also presents data that suggests that bacteria can secrete compounds that can increase the negative charge of cells to which they are attached or bacteria and viruses can cause cells that they infect to secrete compounds that increase the negative charge of the cells. Because immune defense cells, such as NK cells and macrophages, also have a negative charge, these cells are repulsed by the strong negative electrical field of cancer cells when they try to approach these cells (Van Rinsum et al., 1986; Cure, 1995; Acevedo et al., 1998). According to Dr. Acevedo, "Since all the normal cells from our immune system, macrophages, NK cells and B cells, express in their membranes a 'normal' negative charge, the high negative charge of hCG and its subunits demonstrated to be present in the cell membranes of embryonic and fetal cells, in sperm cells in every stage of development, and in all cancer cells irrespective of type or origin as membrane-associated hCG, make all these cells immunologically inert. The cells from the immune system *are restricted from approaching, and adhering to cancer cells*, since negative charges repel. That is the reason why the embryo and fetus, which under normal conditions are 50% foreign to the mother, are able to survive the immune system of the mother, and why sperm cells and cancer cells also survive" (Acevedo, 2002).

Biologically Closed Electric Circuits. The application of electrical currents into cancerous tissue has been found to have a beneficial effect in some cases of cancer. Dr. Björn Nordenström and Dr. Rudolf Pekar have pioneered research where specially-made platinum needles (electrodes) are inserted directly into tumors (Nordenström, 1983; Pekar, 1997). This form of therapy is known as electrochemical therapy because it destroys portions of cancerous tumors by both electrical and chemical means. The needles are connected to an electrical device that produces a direct current. The needles with a positive charge are anodes, while the needles with a negative charge are cathodes. When low voltage (6 to 8 volts) and low micro-amperage (40-80mA) direct currents are administered, the tumor area around the anode becomes highly acidic due to the attraction of negatively-charged chloride ions and the formation of hydrochloric acid (pH 1-2). The tumor areas around the cathode become highly basic (pH 12-14) due to the attraction of positively-charged sodium ions and the formation of sodium hydroxide (Yu-Ling, 1997). Chlorine gas emerges from the skin at entry points of the anodes and hydrogen gas emerges from the entry points of the cathodes (Chou et al., 1997). This strong change in pH is one of the factors involved in killing and injuring tumor cells. *So in a sense, direct current stimulation is a form of pH therapy. We suspect that devices that create electromagnetic fields and current flows in the body all have some effect on intracellular and extracellular pH.* The effectiveness of this type of treatment is dependent on electrode placement and dosage of electrical charge administered in coulombs (Chou et al., 1997). Dr. Yu-Ling reported at Fourth International Symposium on Biologically Closed Electric Circuits that by 1997 over seven thousand cases of malignant tumors had been treated in China by this treatment (Yu-Ling, 1997).

One of Nordenström's techniques is to place the positive electrode into the tumor and the negative electrode outside of the tumor (O'Clock, 1997). This will result in an increased flow of electrons into the tumor, a change in the electrical field around a tumor, and activation of membrane receptors and ion channels. If tumor cells are in fact electron-deficient, this increased flow of electrons, membrane receptor effects, and movement of ions through ion channels will have definite effects on cellular metabolic processes. O'Clock's work has also confirmed Ross Adey's findings that windows of frequency and amplitude exist for tumor cell suppression and proliferation (O'Clock, 1997). The application of direct current to tumor cells has been found to change the membrane potential of tumor cells, nutrient uptake by tumor cells, reduce DNA production by tumor cells, and increase immune activity, particularly the attraction of white blood cells to the tumor site (Chou et al., 1997; Douwes and Szasz, 1997; O'Clock, 1997). The application of direct current causes electrolysis, electrophoresis, electro-osmosis, and electro-poration to occur in biological tissues, creating microenvironmental chemical changes and microelectrical field changes (Li et al., 1997). Changing the membrane potential and membrane permeability of tumor cell membranes with direct current changes both the extracellular and intracellular environment of the tumor cells (Douwes and Szasz, 1997). The chemistry of the microenvironment of healthy cells, injured cells, and cancerous cells and the microelectrical field of these cells are interrelated. *Changes in one results in changes in the other.* This is easier to remember if you understand that all the chemistry of biological organisms involves an exchange of energy. In this type of electrical treatment tumors will destroy some cells by electrolysis and cause other cancer cells to lose their stealth cloaking coating of negatively-charged glycoprotein complexes that have hidden the tumor from the immune system. Loss of this cloaking device allows activation of immune defenses to attack the tumor, including production of cytokines and interferon, and tumor destruction by cytotoxic T-cells and macrophages.

Bacteria and viruses in cancer. Another interesting idea is the concept that bacteria and viruses can change the cell coats of cells and that these infections are associated with certain types of cancer. Back in the 1950s Virginia Livingston-Wheeler promoted the idea that cancers are associated with a particular type of pleomorphic bacteria, which she named "Progenitor cryptocides" (Greek for 'the hidden killer'), after she consistently grew this microbe from cancerous tissues. For detailed information on her work see (Livingston-Wheeler and Wheeler, 1977; Livingston-Wheeler and Addeo, 1984; Cantwell, 1990). Certain types of bacteria are known to colonize areas of the body, particularly areas that have compromised blood supply and regional hypoxia. These bacteria naturally produce biofilms as a way of protecting themselves from the immune system. For example, pseudomonas bacteria can produce a secretion of carbohydrates within which they encapsulate themselves (Straus et al., 1989). These negatively-charged cell coats electrically-repulse attacking immune cells. By attaching themselves to human tissue, it is very likely that these bacteria are using electrical defenses and practicing a natural form of gene therapy. In fact, some researchers are experimenting with the use of anaerobic bacteria as a form of cancer gene therapy. When anaerobic bacteria are injected into the body, they will accumulate in hypoxic tumor areas. If suitably-modified, these bacteria could be engineered to produce anti-malignant proteins as they reproduce (Lemmon et al., 1997). It takes no great stretch of the imagination to conceptualize the ideas that infectious agents could: 1) alter the genetic machinery of the cells to which they are attached, promoting the production of certain proteins and hormones; 2) create biofilms around cells, altering their surface charge and impacting cell mineral concentrations, cell membrane functions, etc.; 3) or secrete their own form of chorionic gonadotropin, which would change the electrical characteristics of the cells to which they are attached. Human chorionic gonadotropin is also a growth factor for certain types of cancer.

After reviewing the papers of Acevedo and Cure, we have formed the opinion that that the presence of hCG on tumor cell surfaces will increase the negative electrical charge of cancer cells. It is well-recognized that cancer cells can produce this hormone, but certain types of tumor-associated bacteria also produce this hormone (Backus and Affronti, 1981). When Virginia Livingston Wheeler reported this same finding back in the early 1970s (Livingston-Wheeler and Livingston, 1974), her findings were dismissed and she was labeled a quack. Acevedo and others have repeatedly shown that some tumor-associated bacteria will produce hCG or components of this hormone. For example, Acevedo and his colleagues in 1987 did immunocytochemical studies using antisera to hCG, and to its alpha- and beta-subunits. They demonstrated the expression of hCG-like material in nine bacterial strains. "Seven of these were isolated from patients with cancer and were definitely identified as Streptococcus faecalis (three strains), Staphylococcus haemolyticus (two strains) and

Staphylococcus epidermidis and Escherichia coli (single strains). The other two strains were cell-wall-deficient (CWD) variants, one identified as Streptococcus bovis, isolated from the blood of a patient with a fever of unknown origin and a possible brain abscess" (Acevedo et al., 1987). Coatings of proteins, glycoproteins, and glycolipids encapsulate many viruses. These viral coats may contain either sialic acid or the enzyme sialidase. If sialic acid predominates, the virus will have a negative charge, but if sialidase predominates, the virus will have a positive charge (Cure, 1995). Either way, many viruses are endowed with electrical charges. If sialidase predominates, the positively-charged virus will be electrically-attracted to the negatively-charged cell surface. An interesting clinical note is that arginine supplementation can activate latent herpes viral infections. Arginine contains a strongly basic guanidine group. It is possible that arginine can enhance the infectivity of certain types of viruses by changing the electrical charge of the virus or cell membranes. Inhibition of the sialidase enzyme will stop the entrance of viruses into cells. This leads to my point that viral inhibition may occur through chemical measures or electronic neutralization. Chicken soup is a well-known remedy for viral infections of the respiratory tract. When chicken soup is prepared without salt, it contains large amounts of free electrons, which can electrically neutralize viruses with positively-charged coats, preventing viral entry into the cells.

Theoretically, electronic microcurrent, infrared, phototherapy devices, homeopathic preparations, and herbal preparations that supply the body with a plethora of free electrons should also exhibit antiviral activity. Treatments that have been reported to disrupt tumor cell coats include pancreatic enzymes (Acevedo et al., 1998), plant enzymes such as bromelain (Nieper, 1996), beta-carotene (Nieper, 1985), heparin (Nieper at al., 1999), and vaccines against HCH (Acevedo et al., 1998; Triozzi and Stevens, 1999).

Treatment Section: Interfaces/nodal points where changes in cellular electrical activity and physiology can be made. Cellular and ECM electric field effects may be enhanced through application of externally-conducted or inductive electric fields. By correcting mineral deficiencies and improper cell location of minerals, by correcting cell membrane abnormalities secondary to dietary deficiencies of essential fatty acids, and imbalances in fatty acid metabolism.

Treatment devices: Microcurrents in biologically-closed electric circuits may be created by 1) Tissue-penetrating magnetic fields from PEMF devices that create magnetic field induction of electric currents in conductive biological structures, 2) direct current and alternating current microcurrent devices applied to the skin by electrodes or into tissues through needles, 3) acupuncture needling, 4) production of a wide band width of electromagnetic energy by multi-wave oscillators, 5) needle implants into tumors with application of DC current, and 6) phototherapy treatments with lasers and LEDS. The use of electrical and phototherapy devices such as lasers and LEDS will change the electric field of the ECM and create current flow both in the ECM and through the cell membrane, depending on the frequency applied. These changing electrical fields will modify the electrical potential of cell membranes, intracellular mineral concentrations, and cellular energy production by affecting the activity of ionic membrane pumps (Liu et al., 1990; Blank, 1992). Modification of the electrical potential of cell membranes can be used to increase the abnormally-low transmembrane potential of cancer cells and injured tissues. Effects that are seen when membrane potential is increased include enhanced cellular energy (ATP) production, increased oxygen uptake, changes in entry of calcium, movement of sodium out of the cell, movement of potassium into the cell, changes in enzyme and biochemical activity, and changes in cellular pH. It appears that modulation of the electric field of the ECM and changing current flows in biologically-closed electric circuits can increase low transmembrane potential, increase the entry of potassium and calcium, increase sodium and water movement out of the cells, reduce intracellular acidity, improve oxygen entry into hypoxic cells, and increase mitochondrial production of ATP through aerobic metabolism. At this time, researchers both promote and warn against the use of electric and magnetic field devices in the treatment of cancer. The history of the electromagnetic treatment of cancer is long and colorful. Because it would require an entire book to fully explore this history, we will limit this discussion to a few points. Back in the early 1920s, George Lakhovsky developed an instrument he called a radio-cellular oscillator, which he used to experiment on geraniums that had been inoculated with cancer (Lakhovsky, 1939). From these experiments, he decided that he could obtain better results if he constructed an apparatus capable of generating an electrostatic field, which would generate a range of frequencies from three meters to infrared (Lakhovsky, 1934). Lakhovsky believed that living organisms are capable of interrelating by receiving and giving off electromagnetic radiations. *Note: If Lakhovsky's theory is correct, then the potential exists for direct energetic communication between living organisms.* Lakhovsky theorized that each cell of the body is characterized by its own unique oscillation. He also believed that one of the essential causes of cancer formation was that cancerous cells were in oscillatory disequilibrium. He believed the way to bring cells that were in disequilibrium back to their normal oscillations was to provide an oscillatory shock (Lakhovsky, 1939). Royal Rife on the other hand believed that oscillatory shock could be used to kill infectious organisms and cancer cells. Either way, changing the oscillation of cancer cells has been thought to be beneficial. Lakhovsky theorized that an instrument that provided a multitude of frequencies would allow every cell to find and vibrate in resonance with its own frequency. In 1931, he invented an instrument called the Multiple Wave Oscillator. Until his death in 1942, he treated and cured a number of cancer patients (Lakhovsky, 1939). Other individuals who have used his MWO have also reported similar results. Individuals such as Royal Rife in the 1930s and Antoine Priore in the 1960s also invented electronic equipment that was reported to benefit patients with cancer (Bearden, 1988). Whether you believe these experiments or not is up to you. But if Lakhovsky, Rife, and Priore were correct, then equipment that addresses and attempts to correct the electrical derangements of cancer cells can be beneficial in some cases.

Polychromatic states and health: a unifying theory? Prigonine's 1967 description of dissipative structures gave a model and an understanding of how open systems, like biological organisms, that have an uninterrupted flow of energy can self-organize. Biological systems are designed to take in and utilize energy from chemical sources (food), but they can also utilize energy and information from resonant interactions with electromagnetic fields and acoustical waves to maintain their dynamic organization. According to Ho, "Energy flow is of no consequence unless the energy is trapped and stored within the system where it circulates before being dissipated" (Ho, 1996). In our opinion, this means that cellular structures that tranduce, store, conduct, and couple energy are critical features of any living organism.

Living systems are characterized by a complex spectrum of coordinated action and rapid intercommunication between all parts (Ho, 1996). The ideal complex activity spectrum of a healthy state is polychromatic, where all frequencies of stored energy in the spectral range are equally represented and utilized (Ho, 1996). In an unhealthy state, some frequencies may be present in excess and other frequencies may be missing. For example, it has been reported that a healthy forest emits a polychromatic spectrum of acoustical frequencies and an unhealthy forest will have holes in its frequency spectrum. Yet when the forest regains its health, it again emits a polychromatic spectrum of frequencies. The frequency holes got filed in. When an area of the body is not properly communicating, it will fall back on its own mode of frequency production, which, according to Mae-Wan Ho, leads to an impoverishment of its frequency spectrum. In looking at the example of cardiac frequency analyzers, it has been discovered that sick individuals have less heart rate variability than healthy individuals. The concept of polychromatism makes sense when you consider phenomena such as the healing effects of sunlight, full spectrum lights, music, tuning forks, chanting, toning, drumming, crystal bowls, sound therapy, prayer, love, the sound of a loved one's voice, essential oils, flower essences, healing touch, multiwave oscillators, and homeopathics. Something or things (frequency or frequencies) that were missing are provided by these treatments. From the consideration of applied frequency technologies, it can be theorized that one aspect of why these consonant technologies work is because they supply frequencies that are missing in the electromagnetic and acoustical spectral emissions of living organisms. When missing frequencies are supplied, they, in a sense, fill gaps in the frequency spectrum of a living organism. Dissonant technologies would identify frequency excesses and pathogenic frequencies and would provide frequency neutralization by phase reversal. Electromagnetic technologies such as Rife and radionics may act by phase reversal and neutralization of pathogenic frequencies. Royal Rife also theorized that his equipment used resonant transmission of energy that caused pathogenic organisms to oscillate to the point of destruction. If we consider polychromatism to be the model of the healthy state, then it makes sense that technologies such as electrodermal screening and voice analysis that detect frequency imbalances (excesses and deficiencies) can play beneficial roles in health care. We believe that in the future, doctors will more widely utilize equipment such as electrodermal screening, acoustical spectrum analyzers, electromagnetic spectral emission analyzers, and their software for diagnostic purposes. This type of equipment can be used to identify and treat frequency imbalances. This discussion ties in such concepts as acupuncture and neural therapy. Acupuncture may help address and remove impedances or blocks to energy mobilization by helping to reconnect disconnected energy pathways back into a coherent and harmonic flow. Neural therapy may act by neutralizing aberrant local signal generators in traumatized and scarred tissue. In a sense, this removes disharmonious music from a particular location. We imagine the application of neural therapy to be like a band conductor correcting a student who is playing out of key.

Ways to support the electrical properties of cells with mineral nutrition and cell membrane repair: In order for cells to operate and control electromagnetic energy and chemical energy production, the cell membranes, which cover the cells and the membranes of cell organelles like the mitochondria and the nucleus, must be healthy and the right minerals must be in the right location and in the right concentrations. Dr. Hans Nieper recognized this fact and he spent his life developing mineral transporters and looking for and using other orthomolecular substances that could support and repair the outer cell membrane and inner membranes of cell organelles.

Optimize membrane structure and function through use of Nieper mineral transporters: The electrical charge of the cell membrane is maintained both by the structure of the membrane and its associated minerals, however these minerals must be in the proper location at the proper concentration for optimization of cellular potential and metabolic activity. Mineral transporters serve the function of special delivery vehicles, placing minerals in optimal cellular and subcellular locations (Alexander, 1997a, 1997b; Nieper et al., 1999). Dr. Nieper found that this approach improved these membranes' natural ability to store electrical charge known as the membrane capacitance function.

Capacitors are well-known electronic components that are composed of two conducting sheets or metal plates separated by a thin layer of insulating material known as a dielectric. Cells contain several forms of biological capacitors, which consist of an insulating material (the membrane) covered on both sides by collections of charged dissolved minerals, which serve the same function as a conducting metal plate. Because the exterior cell membrane and the membranes of cell organelles like the mitochondria in animals and the chloroplasts in plants are biological capacitors they have the capacity to accumulate and store charge and, hence, energy to be given up when needed. Since energy is needed to run any type of machinery, whether mechanical or biological, it makes sense that nutrients that can enhance energy production and energy storage can have profound biological effects.

Improvement in cellular bioenergetics can also be enhanced nutritionally by use of certain nutrients that help provide structural materials for cell membrane repair and facilitation of mitochondrial enzyme production of ATP. Some of the most effective compounds are the mineral transporters amino ethanolphosphates (2-AEPs), orotates, aspartates, and arginates developed by Dr. Hans Nieper. 2- AEP mineral transporters enhance cell membrane capacitance in several ways: first, by repairing damaged cell membranes and second, by effectively delivering minerals to the outer surface of cell membranes. The orotate, aspartate, and arginate mineral transporters are advanced mineral delivery systems that effectively deliver minerals into the interior of cells. Mineral delivery into the cell interior is important because many of the cell's cytoplasmic and mitochondrial enzymes require minerals in order to be activated.

Biological utilization of a mineral encompasses far more than just mineral absorption, including biological utilization of minerals includes mineral absorption, mineral transport in the blood stream, and mineral delivery into the cells. Most mineral supplements generally break apart during the processes of digestion, releasing ionized minerals into the lumen of the digestive tract, which are then moved into the bloodstream. Just getting a mineral into the blood stream doesn't guarantee that the mineral can be directed to any particular tissue or be transported across the cell membrane to the cell interior (Nieper, 1961, 1966a). The joining of carrier molecules with minerals forms electrically-neutral compounds that have different transport properties than unbound ionized minerals (Nieper et al., 1999). Calcium orotate, calcium arginate, calcium aspartate, calcium 2-AEP, magnesium orotate, magnesium arginate, potassium arginate, potassium orotate, potassium-magnesium aspartate, zinc orotate, and zinc aspartate are all mineral transporters. When these mineral transporters are properly manufactured to be acid resistant, they deliver minerals still bound to the transporter into the alkaline environment of the small intestine where the mineral compounds are absorbed relatively intact from the digestive tract into the blood stream with the mineral still bound to the transporter (Alexander, 1997a, 1997b; Nieper et al., 1999). The mineral-transporter complex remains stable in the blood stream with low dissociation, and the minerals are not released until the mineral-transporter complex enters the target tissues/cells. The attachment of minerals to carrier molecules forms electrically neutral stable complexes that allow selective direction of minerals to particular tissues that metabolically use the carrier molecules. This form of directed mineral nutrition even enhances mineral entry even into cells that have disturbed cell membranes. The use of mineral transporters can increase the bioavailability of minerals to injured and cancerous tissue (Nieper, 1966a, 1966b, 1966c, 1967a, 1967b, 1968, 1969, 1970, 1971, 1973, 1985; Buist, 1972, 1978). Dietary correction of essential intracellular mineral deficiencies such as potassium, magnesium, zinc, and other trace elements is also critically important. An example would be the very similar cancer diets promoted by Dr. Hans Nieper or Dr. Max Gerson. Dr. Gerson clinically observed that when cancer patients were responding to treatment, they would lose large amounts of sodium in their urine. This observation was one factor that made him theorize that cancer cells accumulate excess amounts of sodium and water and that the use of a high potassium diet could be very beneficial. Dr. Gerson advised his patients to use a program of natural detoxification that involved a diet containing large amounts of potassium. Gerson used large amounts of fresh vegetable juice and calf liver juice, which provides minerals, enzymes, and electrons to the body. He believed such a diet would also assist in body detoxification, particularly when coffee enemas were used to promote bile flow and bowel cleaning. Cell membrane repair can be initiated by changing the composition of cell membranes with lipid and sterol compounds such as 2-AEP, essential fatty acids, sterols, and phytosterols. According to researchers such as Emanuel Revici, Mary Enig, Hans Nieper, and Patricia Kane, one of the major things that can be done to promote health is to improve membrane structure and membrane functions through nutritional interventions targeted at manipulating lipids, sterols, and minerals. Essential fatty acids, phospholipids, and sterols act as structural components of the cell membrane. Good sources of essential fatty acids and phospholipids are lecithin (phosphatidyl choline) which is found in eggs and soybeans, phosphatidyl serine, flax oil, avocado oil, walnut oil, hazelnut oil, hemp oil, grape seed oil, sesame oil, fish oil, olive oil, evening primrose oil, borage oil, blackcurrant seed oil, butter, coconut oil, and phytosterols. Squalene is a compound found in high concentrations in shark liver oil and, to a lesser degree, in olive oil. Poor choices of fats are cottonseed oil, soybean oil, corn oil, canola oil, transfatty acids, and any hydrogenated or partially hydrogenated oil. *This pretty much eliminates any baked goods created by food manufacturing companies.* 2-AEP is a nutritional supplement usually bound to calcium (calcium 2-AEP) or calcium, magnesium, and potassium (2-AEP complex). 2-AEP is a cell membrane repair molecule that is a precursor of phosphatidyl ethanolamine. 2-AEP helps act as a cell membrane sealant reducing cell entry of toxins and viruses and it helps maintain and improve the electrical potential of cell membranes particularly in cells involved in inflammatory processes (Nieper, 1988). Dr. Nieper reported that people who regularly used AEP mineral transporters along with calcium aspartate or calcium orotate had significantly lower rates of prostate, colon, and breast cancers. Emanuel Revici was an unconventional cancer researcher who developed a treatment for cancer called "guided lipid" therapy. Revici believed cancer patients had two basic patterns of lipid imbalance either an excess of sterols or an excess of fatty acids. He would test his patients in order to determine which pattern that they had, then he would give either fatty acids or sterols to correct the imbalance (Revici, 1961). Patricia Kane has pioneered the use of RBC membrane analysis to determine nutritional adjustments specific for an individual. Mary Enig has written extensively about the role of dietary fats in disease causation and disease prevention. Hans Nieper developed a series of mineral transporters, such as 2-aminoethanol phosphates (AEP's), orotates, arginates, and aspartates, that deliver minerals to specific cellular locations. He also was one of the first doctors to strongly recommend the use of a squalene and a cell membrane repair supplement called AEP. Squalene is a naturally-occurring polyprenyl compound, structurally similar to beta-carotene, which composes up to 70% of the oils in shark livers. Squalene is an important nutritional compound that, in conjunction with AEP, magnesium, zinc, selenium, and the amino acid taurine, can help stabilize the structure and functions of cell membranes. Squalene has a particular role in cancer and degenerative diseases in that, along with AEP, it helps support membrane structure and function. Squalene also has important roles in wound healing, immune system regulation, and the production of steroid hormones. The body's natural production of dhea and pregnenolone can be increased by ingestion of squalene. These steroid hormones are surveillance hormones, having important roles in reducing cancerous transformation in degenerative tissues. Cellular membrane capacitance and cellular energy production may also be enhanced by inductively-created or conducted electric fields in specific *frequency and amplitude (amperage) windows and also by acoustic vibrations.* A cell or body is coupled to an electric field in proportion to its capacitance such that the greater the frequency of the electrical field, the greater the current flow in the cell or body. For soft tissues, low frequency natural or applied electrical fields create currents that are conducted primarily along the surface of cells in the ECM-cell membrane interface. Conduction of electrical currents in the ECM is the dominant effect when very low frequency electrical fields are created in or applied to biological tissues. When high frequency fields are applied with external signal generators, this results in the charging of the cell membranes, causing an increase in cell membrane capacitance and increased conduction of current through the cell membranes. Because cell membranes naturally have capacitance, this makes the cell membrane frequency-dependent conductors. At high frequencies, a greater percentage of current will flow into and out the cell as a circuit loop. Higher frequency fields can strongly affect cell membrane permeability, which in turn can affect nutrient entry into the cells and toxin release from the cells and the ECM. I have done some research with both high frequency multiwave oscillators and experimental whole body phototherapy equipment and I have found that both type I and type II diabetics *will have a fall in blood sugar* when exposed to these devices. *A note of caution: diabetics and cancer patients should only stay in a multiwave oscillator field for 3-5 minutes when they first start because some individuals will have excessive toxin release and a rapid decline in blood sugar.* These individuals need time to clear toxins from their tissue and bloodstream through their organs of elimination. In our experience, phototherapy is gentler and the effects produced, while just as significant, are not as rapid as the effects we have seen with multiwave oscillators. We believe the improvement with glucose control that can be achieved with these types of equipment is related to frequency-induced effects on insulin receptors and cell membrane glucose transport mechanisms. In summary, an increase in cellular membrane capacitance may change membrane permeability, increase cellular nutrient and mineral entry into the cell, and facilitate release of impregnated toxins from the membrane and cell interior.

Addressing genetic issues. The genetic machinery of the cell controls ECM, glyocalyx, cell membrane, cell membrane receptor, and internal cellular macromolecular composition. The genetic machinery of the cell can be altered to an abnormal state by hereditary factors and environmental factors such as viruses, toxic chemicals, heavy metals, radiation, free radical damage, and age-accumulated errors in transcription. Genetic abnormalities include DNA strand breaks, acquired dysfunction of DNA repair mechanisms, mutations in genes that drive the cell to divide, mutations in genes that suppress cell division, and failure to properly code mRNA. If improvements are made in genetic repair and removing genetic toxins, then the types of proteins, lipids, and carbohydrates manufactured by the cell will change. Genetic mutations can by modified by down-regulating oncogenes. Genetic repair can be improved by the use of nutrients such as folic acid and zinc to increase the activity of DNA transcriptase and Vitamin B12, B6, and methionine to improve DNA methylation (Osiecki, 2002). Other strategies can also be used. Dr. Hans Nieper addressed genetic repair by the use of products such as Dionaea muscipula and Iridodial. "Carnivorous plant extracts derived from the Venus Fly-Trap plant contain the active enzymes *endopeptidase* and *endonuclease*. These are special gene-eliminating substances" (Nieper et al., 1999). Venus Fly-Trap plants excrete substances, which extinguish the gene information of ingested insects because otherwise, the absorbed gene information from the insect would possibly go in their own gene system and change it. The carnivorous plant of the "Venus Fly-Trap" contains about a dozen substances, such as *plumbagin*, *droseron*, and *hydroxydroseron*, which extinguish open gene information. According to Dr. Nieper, the extract of Venus Fly-Trap extinguishes genetic replication of malignant cells. This extract is also useful in eliminating tissue damaged by radiation therapy, while leaving normal cells unaffected. Venus Fly-Trap is botanically termed *Dionaea muscipula*.

Iridodials are a primary source of *dialdehydes*, which "are extremely powerful genetic-repair factors" (Nieper et al., 1999). Dialdehydes are "lipid soluble agents that can penetrate the lipid membranes of the outer cells of tumours" (Nieper et al., 1999). Iridodial is extremely similar to the activated dialdehyde, called didrovaltrate. Insects and ants in particular and carnivorous plants are "the most effective producers of gene repair substances" (Nieper, 1990). Insects are, phylogenetically, extremely old. Their ability to conserve and safeguard their gene system is superb. Similar to sharks, they hardly ever develop tumors. They are able to host large amounts of viruses without showing ill effects. Yet insects have *no immune system* – phylogenesis only equipped them with a repair principle called Iridodial (Nieper, 1990). According to Hans Nieper, the aldehydic iridoides (Iridodial) from insects inhibits viruses from causing genetic alterations (Nieper, 1985). These gene-repairing Iridodials work by inactivating the undesired genetic material from an infecting virus, thus protecting the cellular genome. Dr. Peter Thies of Germany first described the anti-malignant, genetic-repair properties of Iridodials in 1985. Also in 1985, Dr. Didier of Gifhorn, Germany first reported pulmonary tumor regression by use of Iridodial (Nieper, 1990).

Dr. Nieper reported that both Dionaea muscipula and Iridodial could extinguish cells, which were genetically-impaired (Nieper, 1996). Therefore, cells that were improperly programmed would be discarded (Nieper, 1984). Such undesired information may otherwise result in the conversion of a normal cell into a cancerous cell. Dr. Nieper found that cells already transformed could be induced to die while normal cells were left unaffected. Gene-repair therapy "represents in many ways, an imitation of the cancer defense of our body" (Nieper, 1985). Dr. Nieper reported that Iridodial and Dionaea muscipula were completely free of any side effects, and so non-toxic that they could be administered without complication in early and suspected stages of the disease for an *unlimited time* (Nieper, 1990). Dr. Hans Nieper believed that Iridodial and Dionaea Muscipula outdistanced most other substances for use in cancer. Dr. Nieper reported that his first choice in his nontoxic approach to cancer was the combined use of the extract of Venus Fly-Trap (Dionaea Muscipula) and the ant extract Iridodial (Nieper, 1990; 1996). Protection of cell membranes, mitochondria, and genetic machinery through the use of exogenous antioxidants and promotion of the production and regeneration of endogenous intracellular and extracellular antioxidant and Redox systems, particularly glutathione pathways. Oxygen is required by the metabolic reactions of our cells that obtain energy from the chemical burning of food. In the process of energy production, some toxic compounds are normally produced. When energy is produced in the mitochondria of cells, some of the oxygen is converted to a variety of free radicals such as superoxide (O2-), hydrogen peroxide (H2O2), and hydroxyl (OH-) radicals. These free radicals are extremely reactive molecules that contain at least one unpaired electron in their outer orbital shell. Body exposure to chemical toxins and radiation also produce free radicals. Unless adequate amounts of cellular and extracellular antioxidants are available, these free radicals will begin to damage cellular structures such as the cell membranes, the mitochondria, the nucleic acids of DNA, and cellular proteins, impairing the ability of the cells to repair themselves and reproduce (Morel et al., 1999). When cell membranes are damaged by free radicals, their ability to hold an electrical charge (capacitance) and their ability to transport minerals and other nutrients is disrupted. When mitochondria are damaged, the cells ability to make energy is impaired. When the genetic code is damaged, cells cannot reproduce normal cells. Free radicals also cause lipid peroxidation, which can result in lowering HDL cholesterol and damage to the cell membranes lining blood vessels. When the delicate membranes lining blood vessels are damaged, an inflammatory process may result which leads to thickening of blood vessels and arterial plaque. The tissue reactions created by free radicals are now thought to be involved in premature aging, cancer, atherosclerosis, arthritis, immune disorders, and other degenerative diseases. The redox status of the cells depends on the concentrations of the oxidized (inactive) and reduced (active) components of the major redox molecules, which act as homeostatic redox buffers. For example, the ratio of oxidized GSSG to reduced GSH reflects the redox status within the cell. In healthy cells, a ration of GSSG/GSH usually averages 1%, which means that the intracellular concentration of GSH is roughly 100 times greater than the intracellular concentration of its oxidized component GSSG. Any change in this ratio will greatly affect the redox status within the cell. When oxidative conditions occur in injury, the oxidized component predominates and genetic activity, cell organelle functions, and cell detoxification functions are impaired.

Providing a source of free electrons: Free radicals result from both natural biochemical processes and environmental factors, such as exposure to chemical toxins, heavy metals, ultraviolet light, x-rays, radiation therapy, nuclear radioactivity, alcohol, and smoking. Because free radicals are defined as molecules that have lost an electron, they can be said to be electron-deficient. These electron-deficient molecules then search the body in any attempt to find a replacement that they can steal, so they can also be thought of as electron thieves. The replacement electrons are generally stolen from cell proteins, cellular DNA, or cell membranes. When enough electrons are taken from these cells, the cells are damaged so that they can then die, undergo cancerous transformation, or be repaired by an antioxidant. Because free radicals are continuously produced as a natural toxic byproduct of energy production, the cells use a variety of antioxidant systems to prevent their accumulation. Antioxidants are life's free radical scavengers. The cellular antioxidants are chemical compounds that have the ability to supply the electron-deficient free radicals with electrons, therefore neutralizing their oxidative destruction of the cells biomolecules. The key element is that antioxidants supply electrons.

From a biologist's point of view, antioxidants are biological chemicals that are able to donate some of their own electrons to neutralize electron-deficient free radicals. Conventional wisdom typically holds that antioxidants have to be nutritive substances, though from a physicist's point of view, antioxidant effects can also be achieved by other methods.

New research has shown that external electronic devices such as microcurrent machines, low power lasers, LEDS, and infrared lamps can also supply electrons. This is the concept of electronic and photonic antioxidants by using physiologically acceptable wavelengths of light (visible and far infrared light) or providing electrical currents in the microcurrent range through application of DC electricity by microcurrent devices. Due to tissue interactions with the photons of light (the photoelectric effect), when light of the right frequency (far infrared or visible light) interacts with biological tissues, electrons are produced. At a fundamental level, a nutrient antioxidant is simply a chemical carrier of extra electrons and the same effect of providing extra electrons by chemical means can be also achieved by exposure to the photons of far infrared or visible light. Far infrared and visible light are bands of electromagnetic energy which are particularly acceptable and beneficial to living creatures. This photonic antioxidant effect provides part of the explanation of how the "vital rays" of far infrared and visible light are involved in healing.

In addition the use of these devices in this way, they also help reestablish biocurrent flow in electrically resistive tissue, reducing the resistance of the cancerous tissue and facilitating a more normal capacitance. Warning: microcurrents and PEMF devices should not be used on pregnant women or people with pacemakers.

Microcurrent electrical therapy and PEMF therapy: Microcurrent devices deliver weak electrical currents directly to the tissues through the use of needle implants or attached electrodes. A PEMF device applies a magnetic field to the body, which *induces the production* of weak electrical currents in the tissues. As previously stated, these weak biocurrents can influence the flow of blood and oxygen to the tissues and the flow of ions and of nutrients into the cells. This enhancement of circulation and nutrient exchange can be beneficial in improving cellular bioenergetics. Doctors, chiropractors, dentists, physical therapists, and other practitioners currently use microcurrent electrotherapy for a variety of clinical conditions. In fact, it is a rapid treatment for many pain-related disorders because it can provide fast relief of symptoms and promote faster tissue healing. The advantages of microcurrent electrotherapy are multiple. It has significantly fewer side-effects than drugs. In many cases, it can give symptom relief in mere minutes and it supports cellular repair processes, unlike many pharmacological agents that can have toxic effects when used long-term for chronic conditions. The first modern acceptable electrotherapy devices to receive wide medical utilization were transcutaneous nerve stimulation devices called TENS units. TENS devices use a small current of electricity in the milliamp range at low frequencies – typically eight cycles per second or less to block the body's ability to perceive the pain (Leo et al., 1986). TENS devices are believed to stimulate A-beta pain-suppressing nerve fibers to overwhelm chronic pain-carrying C fibers and to release endorphins (Melzack and Wall, 1965; Mercola and Kirsch, 1995). According to Dr. Mercola, for TENS devices to be effective, they require that the current be strong enough to be felt. "Patients are advised to set the current at the maximum comfortable tolerance, but the nervous system gradually accommodates to this high level of current, causing tolerance similar to that of chemical analgesics. Increasing the current causes mild electrical burns in about one third of the patients. The technique provides no significant residual effect" (Mercola and Kirsch, 1995). Microcurrent devices use a current of lower intensity in the microampere range with a longer pulse width. The currents that microcurrent devices use are 1000 times less than milliampere range of TENS with pulse widths 2500 times longer than the pulse in a typical TENS unit (Mercola and Kirsch, 1995).

Unlike TENS devices, microcurrent devices help stimulate cellular and tissue repair processes by using electrical currents in the physiological range used by the body. Administration of electric currents in physiologic ranges by microcurrent devices have a number of advantageous cellular effects including the increase of ATP generation by almost 500%, enhancement of amino acid transport through the cell membranes, and increasing cellular protein synthesis (Cheng et al., 1986). It is also likely that cell membrane transport of minerals is also enhanced because microcurrent devices help correct the reduced cellular capacitance of damaged cells and increase the reduced electrical conductance of injured tissue. Injured tissue begins to heal faster when cellular energy production increases, the cells regain normal capacitance, and the tissues regain normal conduction of electrical currents (Becker, 1985; Vodovnik and Karba, 1992), allowing reestablishment of normal communication with the rest of the body through the liquid crystal connective tissue communication system (Ho, 1998).

Ensure Adequate Hydration

One can initiate autorepair mechanisms by removal of energetic blockages (acupuncture, homeopathy, neural therapy, infrared emitters, phototherapy devices, microcurrent devices, pulsed electromagnetic field devices, etc.) and detoxify toxic chemicals and heavy metals in the ECM by massage, oral, and IV chelation, infrasonic devices, ultrasonic devices, infrared devices, phototherapy devices, and microcurrent devices. Many clinicians use detoxification strategies that mobilize toxins and promote excretion through skin (infrared saunas), liver-GI tract, and kidneys. Improving cellular oxygen levels by opening up the microcirculation with enzymes like bromelain, papain, pancreatin, nattokinase, and oral and IV EDTA.

Increasing tissue oxygen levels with ozone therapy and hyperbaric oxygen. Change the composition of the ECM/glycocalyx/cell membrane interface with compounds like glyconutrients that help change the composition and charge of proteoglycans and the composition and activity of cell receptors. Possible nutrients include Betaglucans, IP-6, Aloe vera extracts, arabinogalactans, glucosamine, polysaccharides derived from mushrooms, and alginates.

Use of cell therapy. Cell therapy may be provided orally or by implantation. Active cell therapy research is now taking place with the implantation of stem cells such as mesenchymal cells, which can differentiate into osteoblasts, chondroblasts, myoblasts, and fibroblasts. Cell therapy is also available with oral glandular products that provide organ-specific components. These organ specific components supply a unique form of nutrition to organ cells that is different from oral and IV nutrient programs. Cell therapy can help balance hormone production by the endocrine glands when a preexisting endocrine deficiency exists.

In closing the goals to work toward in electronic cancer nutrition: 1) Intervene nutritionally at the level of the ECM-glycocalyx-cell membrane level with enzymes, 2) Repair cell membranes and cell membrane potential with proper selections of fats, sterols, phytosterols, AEP, squalene, and mineral transporters, 3) Improve cell signaling mechanisms (role of glyconutrients), 4) Correct imbalances in intracellular minerals that are needed for maintenance of cell membrane capacitance and enzyme cofactors by utilizing mineral transporters, 5) Correct DNA breaks and DNA repair mechanisms with gene support nutrients, vitamin B12, B6, folic acid, cell therapy implants, gene repair extracts (Dionaea muscipula and Iridodial), 6) Improve macromolecular production, utilization and secretion of proteins (enzymes and structural proteins), peptide (hormones, growth factors, growth inhibitors, and cytokines), lipids, and carbohydrates (energy source and signaling molecules), 7) Improve intracellular energy production with vitamins, carnitine, coenzyme Q10, intracellular mineral transporters, 8) Correct pH alterations with diet, 9) Facilitate antioxidant functions, 10) Facilitate detoxification of the ECM and intracellular compartments.

References

Acevedo HF. Human chorionic gonadotropin (hCG), the hormone of life and death: a review. *J Exp Ther Oncol* 2002 May-Jun; 2(3):133-45.

Acevedo HF, Pardo M, Campbell-Acevedo E, Domingue GJ. Human choriogonadotropin-like material in bacteria of different species: electron microscopy and immunocytochemical studies with monoclonal and polyclonal antibodies. *J Gen Microbiol* 1987 Mar; 133 (Pt 3):783-91.

Acevedo HF, Tong JY, Hartsock RJ. Human chorionic gonadotropin-beta subunit gene expression in cultured human fetal and cancer cells of different types and origins. *Cancer* 1995 Oct 15; 76(8):1467-75.

Acevedo H, Gonzalez N, Moss R. Trophoblastic Hormones and Cancer: A Breakthrough in Treatment? Comprehensive Cancer Care Conference, Session 205: June 13, 1998. *http://www.cmbm.org/conferences/ccc98/transcripts/205.html.*

Adey WR. Tissue interactions with nonionizing electromagnetic fields. *Physiol Rev* 1981; 61:435-514.

Adey WR. Physiological signaling across cell membranes and cooperative influences of extremely low frequency electromagnetic fields. In: *Biological Coherence and Response to External Stimuli*, H. Frohlich, ed., Heidelberg, Springer-Verlag, pgs 148-170, 1988.

Adey WR. ELF magnetic fields and promotion of cancer: experimental studies. In *Interaction Mechanisms of low-level Electromagnetic Fields in Living Systems,* (eds. B. Norden and C. Ramel). Oxford, England: Oxford University Press, pgs 23-46, 1992.

Adey WR. Electromagnetics in biology and medicine. In *Modern Radio Science*, (ed. H. Matsumoto). Oxford, England: Oxford University Press, pgs 277-245, 1993.

Aidley DJ, Stanfield PR. *Ion Channels: Molecules in Action.* Cambridge, UK: Cambridge University Press, 1996.

Alexander AD. The healthy cell: Its structure and functions that are so essential to disease prevention and treatment. *INI Newsletter* June 1997a.

Alexander AD. Calcium 2-AEP and calcium orotate found essential in the prevention and treatment of osteoporosis. *INI Newsletter* June 1997b.

Ambrose EJ, James AM, Lowick JHB. Differences between the electrical charge carried by normal and homologous tumor cells. *Nature* 1969; 177:576-577.

Atema A, Buurman KJ, Noteboom E, Smets LA. Potentiation of DNA adduct formation and cytotoxicity of platinum-containing drugs by low pH. *Int J Cancer* 1993; 54:166–172.

Backus BT, Affronti LF. Tumor-associated bacteria capable of producing a human choriogonadotropin-like substance. *Infect Immun* 1981 Jun; 32(3):1211-5.

Beal JB. Biosystems liquid crystals & potential effects of natural & artificial electromagnetic fields (EMFs) 1996. Website: http://frontpage.simnet.is/vgv/jim1.htm

Bearden TE. *AIDS Biological Warfare*. Greenville, TX: Tesla Book Company, 1988.

Becker RO. The bioelectric factors in amphibian limb regeneration. *Journal of Bone and Joint Surgery* 1961; 43A:643-656.

Becker RO. The electrical control of growth processes. *Medical Times* 1967; 95: 657-669.

Becker RO, Murray DG. The electrical control system regulating fracture healing in amphibians. *Clin Orthop Rel Res* 1970; 73:169.

Becker RO. Stimulation of partial limb regeneration in rats. *Nature* 1972; 235:109- 111.

Becker RO. The basic biological data transmission and control system influenced by electrical forces. *Ann N Y Acad Sci* 1974; 238: 236-241.

Becker RO. *Cross Currents*. London, England: Bloomsbury Publishing, 1990.

Becker RO, Selden G. *The Body Electric*. New York: W. Morrow and Company Inc, 1985.

Becker RO, Bassett CAL, Bachman CH. Bioelectric factors controlling bone structure. In: *Bone Biodynamics*, ed. H. Frost. New York: Little Brown, 1964.

Bender DA. *Introduction to Nutrition and Metabolism, 3rd ed.* New York, New York: Taylor and Francis Inc., 2002.

Blad B, Baldetorp B. Impedance spectra of tumour tissue in comparison with normal tissue: A possible clinical application for electrical impedance tomography. *Physiological Measurement* 17 Suppl 4A:A105-115, 1996.

Blank M. Na, K -ATPase function in alternating electric fields, *FASEB J* 1992; 6:2434-2438.

Board M, et al. High Km glucose-phosphorylating (glucokinase) activities in a range of tumor cell lines and inhibition of rates of tumor growth by the specific enzyme inhibitor mannoheptulose. *Cancer Res* 1995 Aug 1; 55(15):3278-85.

Borgens RB, Robinson KR, Vanable JW, McGinnis ME. *Electric Fields In Vertebrate Repair.* NY: Alan R. Liss, 1989.

Brewer AK, Passwater R. Physics of the cell membrane. Mechanisms involved in cancer. *Am Lab* 1976 April; 10; 37-45.

Brewer AK. *High pH Cancer Therapy with Cesium.* Published by The A. Keith Brewer International Science Library, 325 N. Central Avenue, Richland Center, Wisconsin 53581. Phone # 608-647-6513. email – drbrewer@mwt.net, 1985.

Brighton CT, Black J, Pollack SR. *Electrical Properties of Bone and Cartilage* New York: Grune & Stratton, 1979.

Brown G. *The Energy of Life: The Science of What Makes Our Minds and Bodies Work.* New York, NY: The Free Press, 1999.

Buist R. *Biological Applications of Orotates: Orotates Mineral Salts of Vitamin B13.* Sydney: Colprint Press, 1972.

Buist R. Orotates: *The Ultimate in Mineral Transportation.* Sydney: Colprint Press, 1978.

Cantwell AR Jr. *The Cancer Microbe: The Hidden Killer in Cancer, AIDS, and Other Immune Diseases.* Los Angeles: Aries Rising Press, 1990.

Charman RA. Electrical Properties of Cells and Tissues. In *Clayton's Electrotherapy 10th edition* (eds. S. Kitchen and S. Bazin), London, UK: WB Saunders Company Ltd., 1996.

Cheng N, Van Hoff H, Bockx E, et al. The effect of electric currents on ATP generation protein synthesis, and membrane transport in rat skin. *Clin Orthop* 1982; 171:264-72.

Chou CK, Vora N, Li JR, et al. Development of electrochemical treatment at the City of Hope. In *Proceedings of the Fourth International Symposium on Biologically Closed Electric Circuits.* Bloomington, MN: International Association for Biologically Closed Electric Circuits in Biomedicine, pgs 100-103, October 26-29, 1997.

Cone CD. Variation of the transmembrane potential level as a basic mechanism of mitosis control. *Oncology* 1970; 24:438-470.

Cone CD. The role of surface electrical transmembrane potential in normal and malignant mitogenesis. *Ann NY Acad Sci* 1975; 238:420-35.

Cone CD. *Transmembrane Potentials and Characteristics of Immune and TumorCells.*

Cope FW. A medical application of the Ling Association-Induction Hypothesis: The high potassium, low sodium diet of the Gerson cancer therapy. *Physiol Chem Phys* 1978; 10(5):465-468.

Cure JC. Cancer an electrical phenomenon. *Resonant* 1991; 1(1).

Cure JC. On the electrical characteristics of cancer. Paper presented at the *Second International Congress of Electrochemical Treatment of Cancer*. Jupiter, Florida: October 1995.

Dang CV, Lewis BC, Dolde C, et al. Oncogenes in tumor metabolism, tumorigenesis, and apoptosis. *J Bioenerg Biomembr* 1997; 29:345–354.

Douwes FR, Szasz A. Electrochemical therapy of cancer. A new treatment modality for cancer destruction. Clinical use and experience. *Proceedings of the Fourth International Symposium on Biologically Closed Electric Circuits.* Bloomington, MN: International Association for Biologically Closed Electric Circuits in Biomedicine, pgs 75-99, October 26-29, 1997.

Eckert KA, Kunkel TA. Fidelity of DNA synthesis catalyzed by human DNA polymerase and HIV-1 reverse transcriptase: effect of reaction pH. *Nucleic Acids Res* 1993; 21:5212–5220.

Edwards SL. Hypovolaemia: pathophysiology and management options. *Nursing in Critical Care* 1998; 3(2):73-82.

Foster KR, Schepps JL. Dielectric properties of tumor and normal tissues at radio through microwave frequencies. *J Microwave Power* 1981; 16:107-119.

Fricke H, Morse S. The electric capacity of tumors of the breast. *J Cancer Res* 1926; 10: 340-376.

Frohlich H., ed. *Biological Coherence and Response to External Stimuli.* Heidelberg: Springer-Verlag, 1988.

Fukada E, Yasuda I. On the piezoelectric effect in bone. *J Physiol Soc Japan* 957; 12:1198.

Fukada E. Piezoelectricity of natural biomaterials. *Ferroelectrics* 1984; 60:285-296.

Garnett M. *First Pulse: A Personal Journey in Cancer Research.* New York, NY: first Pulse Projects, 1998.

Garnett M. *Does DNA have a pulse?* Garnett McKeen Laboratory, Inc. 150 Islip Ave. Suite 6, Islip, New York 11751, 2000.

Garnett M, Remo JL. DNA Reductase: A Synthetic Enzyme with Opportunistic Clinical Activity Against Radiation Sickness. *International Symposium on Applications of Enzymes in Chemical and Biological Defense*, Orlando, Florida, May, 2001, p. 41.

Garnett M, Remo JL, Krishnan CV. *Developmental electronic pathways and carcinogenesis.* Garnett McKeen Laboratory, Inc. 150 Islip Ave. Suite 6, Islip, New York 11751. http://www.polymva survivors.com/research_articles.html, 2002.

Gerweck LE. Modification of cell lethality at elevated temperatures: the pH effect. *Radiat Res* 1977; 70:224–235.

Gold J. Proposed treatment of cancer by inhibition of gluconeogenesis. *Oncology* 1968; 22:185-207.

Gold J. Inhibition of gluconeogenesis at the phosphoenolpyruvate carboxykinase and pyruvate carboxylase reactions, as a means of cancer chemotherapy. *Oncology* 1974; 29:74-89.

Gold J. Anabolic profiles in late-stage cancer patients responsive to hydrazine sulfate. *Nutr Cancer* 1981; 3(1):13-9.

Goldin EM, Leeper DB. The effect of low pH on thermotolerance induction using fractionated 45 degrees C hyperthermia. *Radiat Res* 1981; 85:472–479.

Graeber TG, Osmanian C, Jacks T, et al. Hypoxia-mediated selection of cells with diminished apoptotic potential in solid tumours. *Nature* 1999; 379:88–91.

Gray LH, Conger AD, Ebert M, Hornsey S, Scott OC. Concentration of oxygen dissolved in tissues at the time of irradiation as a factor in radiotherapy. *Brit J Radiol* 1953; 26:638-648.

Hakomori SI. Biochemical basis of tumor-associated carbohydrate antigens. Current trends, future perspectives, and clinical applications. *Immunol Allergy Clin North Am* 1990; 10:781–802.

Haltiwanger SG. Clinical use of mineral transporters and their effects on cellmembrane capacitance: *Second International Congress of BioEnergetic Medicine*, Institute of Quantum and Molecular Medicine, February 20-22, 1998.

Hasan NM, Adams GE, Joiner MC, Marshall JF, Hart IR. Hypoxia facilitates tumour cell detachment by reducing expression of surface adhesion molecules and adhesion to extracellular matrices without loss of cell viability. *Br J Cancer* 1998; 77(11):1799-805.

Hazelwood CK, Chang DC, Nichold BJ, Woesner DE. Nuclear magnetic resonance transverse relaxation times of water protons in skeletal muscle. *Biophys J* 1974; 14:583-606.

Hille B. *Ionic Channels of Excitable Membranes 2nd ed.* Sunderland, MA: Sinauer Assoc., 1992.

Ho MW. Bioenergetics and Biocommunication. In *Computation in Cellular and Molecular Biological Systems* (eds., R Cuthbertson, M Holcombe, R Patton). Singapore: World Scientific pgs. 251-264, 1996.

Ho MW. *The Rainbow and the Worm: The Physics of Organisms, 2nd ed.* River Edge, NJ: World Scientific, 1998.

Holash J, Maisonpierre PC, Compton D, et al. Vessel cooption, regression, and growth in tumors mediated by angiopoietins and VEGF. *Science* 1999; 283:1994–1998.

Ivorra A. Bioimpedance Monitoring for physicians: van overview. July, 2002. Website:http://www.cnm.es/~mtrans/PDF's/Bioimpedance_for_physicians_rev1.PDF

Kim JH, Kim SH, Alferi A, et al. Quercitin an inhibitor of lactate transport and hyperthermic sensitizer of hela cells. *Cancer Res* 1984; 44(1):102-6.

Kuin A, Aalders M, Lamfers M, et al. Potentiation of anti-cancer drug activity at low intratumoral pH induced by the mitochondrial inhibitor m-iodobenzylguanidine (MIBG) and its analogue benzylguanidine (BG). *Br J Cancer* 1999; 79:793–801.

Lakhovsky G. Apparatus with circuits oscillating under multiple wavelengths. *U.S. Patent No. 1, 962, 565.* June 12, 1934.

Lakhovsky G. *The Secret of Life: Electricity, Radiation and Your Body.* Translated by M. Clement, London: Heinemann, 1939.

Leeper DB, et al. Effect of i.v. glucose versus combined i.v. plus oral glucose on human tumor extracellular pH for potential sensitization to thermoradiotherapy. *Int J Hyperthermia* 1998 May-Jun; 14(3):257-69.

Lemmon MJ, van Zijl P, Fox ME, et al. Anaerobic bacteria as a gene delivery system that is controlled by the tumor microenvironment. *Gene Ther* 1997; 4(8):791-6.

Leo KC, Dostal WF, Bossen DG, et al. Effect of transcutaneous electrical nerve stimulation characteristics on clinical pain. *Physical Therapy* 1986; 6:200-205.

Li KH, Xin YL, Gu B, et al. Effects of direct electric current on dog liver:possible mechanisms for tumor electrochemical treatment. *Bioelectromagnetics* 1997; 18:2.

Li XQ, Yan YJ. *Electrical transport through individual DNA molecules.* Department of Chemistry, Hong Kong University of Science and Technology, Kowloon, Hong Kong March 30, 2001.

Liboff AR. Electric-field ion cyclotron resonance. *Bioelectromagnetics* 1997; 18(1):85-87.

Ling GN. The Association-Induction Hypothesis: A theoretical foundation provided for the possible beneficial effects of a low sodium, high potassium diet and other similar regimens in the treatment of patients suffering from debilitating illnesses. *Agressologie* 1983; 24(7):293-302.

Ling GN, Ochsenfeld MM. Na+ and K+ levels in living cells: Do they depend on the rate of outward transport of Na+? *Physiol Chem Phys* 1976; 8:389.

Ling GN. *Life at the Cell and Below-Cell Level. The Hidden History of a Fundamental Revolution in Biology.* New York: Pacific Press, 2001.

Liu DS, Astumian RD, Tsong TY. Activation of Na+ and K+ pumping modes of (Na-K)-ATPase by an oscillating electric field. *The Joumal of Biological Chemistry* 1990; 265(13):7260-7267.

Livingston-Wheeler VWC, Livingston AM. Some cultural, immunological, and biochemical properties of Progenitor cryptocides. *Trans N Y Acad Sci* 1974 Jun; 36(6):569-82.

Livingston-Wheeler VWC, Wheeler OW: *The Microbiology of Cancer.* San Diego: Livingston Wheeler Medical Clinic Publication, 1977.

Livingston-Wheeler VWC, Addeo KG: *The Conquest of Cancer.* New York: FranklinWatts Publisher, 1984.

Mahnensmith RL, Aronson PS. The plasma membrane sodium-hydrogen exchanger and its role in physiological and pathophysiological processes. *Circ Res* 1985; 56(6):773-788.

Marieb EN. *Human Anatomy and Physiology* Fourth edition. Redwood City: The Benjamin/Cummings Publishing Company, 1998.

Melzack R, Wall P. Pain mechanisms: a new theory. *Science* 1965; 150:971.

Mercola JM, Kirsch DL. The basis for micro current electrical therapy in conventional medical practice. *Journal of Advancement in Medicine* 1995; 8(2).

Modica-Napolitano J, Singh KK. Mitochondria as targets for detection and treatment of cancer. [http://www-ermm.cbcu.cam.ac.uk/02004453h.htm] *Expert Reviews in Molecular Medicine* April 11, 2001.

Morel Y, Barouki R. Repression of gene expression by oxidative stress. *Biochem J* 1999; 342:481–496.

Moulder JE, Rockwell S. Tumor hypoxia: its impact on cancer therapy. *Cancer Metastasis Rev* 1987; 5:313–341.

Nelson WC. Electrical reactance and its correlates in biological systems: electrophysiological reactivity. Budapest, Hungary, 1995. http://www.energeticmedicine.net/research/xeriod2.doc.

Newell K, Franchi A, Pouyssegur J, et al. Studies with glycolysis-deficient cells suggest that the production of lactic acid is not the only cause of tumor acidity. *Proc Natl Acad Sci* 1993; 90:1127-31.

Nieper H A. Experimental bases and clinical use of electrolyte carrier compounds. *Arztl Forsch* 1961; 15: 510-514.

Nieper HA, Blumberger K. Electrolyte transport therapy of cardiovascular disease in: *Electrolytes and cardiovascular disease*. Ed. Bajusz E. Vol 2: 141-173, Basel/ New York: S. Karger, 1966a.

Nieper HA. *Experimentation clinque de transporteurs de calcium*. 1966b; 7(6): 623-639.

Nieper HA. Clinical experimentation with calcium transport agents. Calcium DL, L-aspartate and calcium-aminoethyl phosphate, 2 powerful anti-inflammatory and antiallergic agents. *Agressologie* 1966c Nov; 7(6):623-639.

Nieper HA. A clinical study of Ca-2-aminoethanolphosphate (2nd communication). *Aggressologie* 1967a; 7(4):4-16.

Nieper HA. A clinical study of the calcium transport substances Ca-l, dl-aspartate and Ca-2-aminoethenol phosphate as potent agents against autoimmunity and other anticytologial aggressions. *Aggressologie* 1967b; 8(4):395-406.

Nieper HA. Comparative study of the clinical effect of dl- asparate (calciretard), of ca-2-calcium aminoethanol phosphate (Ca-EAP) and of the cortisones. *Aggressologie* 1968; 9(3):471-475.

Nieper HA. The anti-inflammatory and immune-inhibiting effects of calcium orotate on bradythropic tissues. *Agressolgie* 1969; 10(4):349-357.

Nieper HA. Recalcification of bone metastases by calcium- diorotate. *Aggressologie* 1970; 11(6):495-503.

Nieper HA. Therapeutically effective calcium diorotate *US Patent 3, 621, 024*, filed Nov. 13, 1968, pat. Nov. 16, 1971.

Nieper HA The clinical effect of calcium- diorotate on cartilaginous tissue, the specific function dependent upon the pentose- metabolism of bradytrophic tissue. *Geriatrie* 1973; 3(4): 82-89.

Nieper HA. Dionaea muscipula (Venus Fly-Trap) Therapy - Excerpt from his lecture at the *Health by Choice Conference*, Atlanta, Georgia, April 1984.

Nieper HA. Genetic repair including 'Iridodial' an insect derived genetic repair factor of important antimalignant effect" *Raum & Zeit* (German Magazine, *Space & Time*), 1990.

Nieper HA. Modern medical cancer therapy following the decline of toxic chemotherapy. *Townsend Letter for Doctors & Patients*, November 1996.

Nordenström BEW. *Biologically Closed Circuits: Clinical, Experience and Theoretical Evidence for an Additional Circulation.* Stockholm, Sweden: Nordic Medical Publications, 1983.

Nuccitelli R. The Involvement of transcellular ion currents and electric fields in pattern formation. In: *Pattern Formation*, (eds. GM Malacinski, SV Bryant), NY: Macmillan Publishing Co., 1984.

O'Clock GD. The effects of in vitro electrical stimulation on normal and malignant eukaryotic cells. In *Proceedings of the Fourth International Symposium on Biologically Closed Electric Circuits.* Bloomington, MN: International Association for Biologically Closed Electric Circuits in Biomedicine, pgs 105-113, October 26-29, 1997.

Ojugo A SE, McSheehy PMJ, McIntyre DJO, et al. Measurement of the extracellular pH of solid tumours in mice by magnetic resonance spectroscopy: a comparison of exogenous 19F and 31P probes. *NMR Biomed* 1999; 12: 495-504.

Oschman JL. *Energy Medicine: The Scientific Basis.* Edinburgh, England: Churchill Livingstone, 2000.

Osiecki H. *Cancer: A Nutritional/Biochemical Approach.* Eagle Farm, Australia: Bioconcepts publishing, 2002.

Pekar R. *Percutaneous Bio-Electrotherapy of Cancerous Tumours: A Documentation of Basic Principles and Experiences with Bio-Electrotherapy.* Munich, Germany: Verlag Wilhelm Maudrich, 1997.

Presman AS. *Electromagnetic Fields and Life.* New York, NY: Plenum Press, 1970.

Regelson W. The 'Grand Conspiracy' against the cancer cure. *Journal of the American Medical Association* 1980; 243(4):337.

Reichart LF. Extracellular matrix molecules. In: *Guidebook to the Extracellular Matrix, Anchor, and Adhesion Proteins,* (ed. T. Kreis and R. Vale). Oxford, England: Oxford University Press, pgs. 335-344, 1999.

Reilly JP. *Applied Bioelectricity: From Electrical Stimulation to Electropathology.* New York: Springer, 1998.

Reynolds TY, Rockwell S, Glazer PM. Genetic instability induced by the tumor microenvironment. *Cancer Res* 1996; 56:5754–5757.

Revici E. *Research in Pathophysiology as Basis for Guided Chemotherapy, with Special Application to Cancer.* Princeton, NJ: D. Van Nostrand Company, 1961.

Rockwell S. Use of hypoxia-directed drugs in the therapy of solid tumors. *Semin Oncol* 1992; 19:29–40.

Rofstad EK. Microenvironment-induced cancer metastasis. *Int J Radiat Biol* 2000; 76:589–605.

Rossi-Fanelli F, et al. Abnormal substrate metabolism and nutritional strategies in cancer management. *JPEN J Parenter Enteral Nutr* 1991 Nov- Dec; 15(6):680-3.

Sartori HE. Cesium therapy in cancer patients. *Phar Biochem and Behavior* 1984; 21(1):11-13.

Scharfetter H. *Structural modeling for impedance-based non-invasive diagnostic methods.* Graz: Thesis for the habilitation at the Faculty of Electrical Engineering Technical University Graz, November 1999.

Schaubel MK, Habal MB. Electropotentials of surgical specimens. *Arch Pathol* 1970; 90:411-415.

Seeger PG, Wolz S. *Successful Biological Control of Cancer: By Combat Against the Causes*. Gesamtherstellung: Neuwieder Verlagsgesellschaft mbH, 1990.

Semenza GL. Involvement of hypoxia-inducible factor 1 in human cancer. *Intern Med* 2002; 41:79-83.

Skarsgard LD, Skwarchuk MW, Vomczan A, et al. The cytotoxicity of melphalan and its relationship to pH, hypoxia and drug uptake. *Anticancer Res* 1995; 15:219–223.

Sharp MG, Adams SM, Walker RA, Brammer WJ, Varley JM. Differential expression of the mitochondrial gene cytochrome oxidase II in benign and malignant breast tissue. *J Pathol* 1992, 168:163-168.

Smith C, Best S. *Electromagnetic Man.* New York: St. Martin's Press, 1989.

Stanish W. The use of electricity in ligament and tendon repair. *Physician Sports Med* 1985; 13:108-116.

Stern RG. Carcinogenesis and the plasma membrane. *Med Hypotheses* 1999 May; 52(5):367-372.

Straus DC, Lonon MK, Woods DE, Garner CW. Production of an extracellular toxic complex by various strains of Pseudomonas cepacia. *J Med Microbiol* 1989 Sep; 30(1):17-22.

Stipanuk MA. *Biochemical and Physiological Aspects of Human Nutrition.* Philadelphia, Pennsylvania: W. B. Saunders Company, 2000.

Stubbs M, Rodrigues L, Howe FA, et al. Metabolic consequences of a reversed pH gradient in rat tumours. *Cancer Res* 1994; 54:4011-4016.

Szent-Gyorgyi A. *Bioelectronics. A Study in Cellular Regulations, Defense, and Cancer.* London: Academic Press, 1968.

Teicher BA. Hypoxia and drug resistance. *Cancer Metastasis Rev* 1994; 13:139–168.

Triozzi PL, Stevens VC. Human chorionic gonadotropin as a target for cancer vaccines [review]. *Oncology Rep* 1999; 6:7–17.

Tsong TY. Deciphering the language of cells. *Trends in Biochemical Sciences* 1989; 14:89-92

Van der Merwe SA, Van den Berg AP, Kroon BB, et al. Modification of human tumour and normal tissue pH during hyperthermic and normothermic antiblastic regional isolation perfusion for malignant melanoma: a pilot study. *Int J Hyperthermia* 1993; 9:205–217.

Van der Zee J, Van der Berg APBroekmeyer-Reurink MP. Temperature and pH during hyperthermic perfusion (meeting abstract). *Thirty-seventh Annual Meeting of the Radiation Research Society.* Seattle, Washington, 1989 March 18-23: page 105.

Van Rinsum J, Smets LA, Van Rooy H, Van Den Eunden DH. Specific inhibition of human natural killer cell-mediated cytotoxicity by sialic acid and sialo-oligosaccharides. *Int J Cancer* 1986; 38:915-22.

Van Winkle LJ. *Biomembrane Transport.* San Diego, California: Academic Press, 1999.

Vaupel P, Schlenger K, Knoop C, Hockel M. Oxygenation of human tumors: evaluation of tissue oxygen distribution in breast cancers by computerized O2 tension measurements. *Cancer Res* 1991; 51(12):3316-22.

Vodovnik L, Karba R. Treatment of chronic wounds by means of electric and electromagnetic fields. A literature review. *Med Bio Engineer Compute* 1992; 30:257-266.

Volk T, et al. pH in human tumor xenografts: effect of intravenous administration of glucose. *Br J Cancer* 1993 Sep; 68(3):492-500.

Von Ardenne M. Principles and concept 1993 of the Systemic Cancer Multistep Therapy (SCMT). Extreme whole-body hyperthermia using the infrared-A technique IRATHERM 2000 -- selective thermosensitisation by hyperglycemia -- circulatory back-up by adapted hyperoxemia. *Strahlenther Onkol* 1994 Oct; 170(10):581-9.

Warburg O. *The metabolism of tumors*. London, England: Constable, 1930.

Warburg O. On the origin of cancer cells. *Science* 1956 Feb; 123:309-14.

Warren L, Fuhrer JP, Buck CA. Surface glycoproteins of normal and transformed cells: a difference determined by sialic acid and a growth-dependent sialyl transferase. *Proc Natl Acad Sci USA* 1972; 69:1838–1842.

Wolfe SL. *Molecular and Cellular Biology.* Belmont, California: Wadsworth Publishing Company, 1993.

Webb SD, Sherratt JA, Fish RG. Mathematical modelling of tumour acidity: regulation of intracellular pH. *J Theor Biol* 1999; 196:237-250.

Weinhouse S. The Warburg hypothesis fifty years later. *Z Krebsforsch Klin Onkol Cancer Res Clin Oncol* 1976; 87:115–126.

Wike-Hooley JL, Haveman J, Reinhold HS. The relevance of tumour pH to the treatment of malignant disease. *Radiother Oncol* 1984; 2:343–366.

Wing T. Modern low voltage microcurrent stimulation: A comprehensive overview. *Chiropractic Economics* 1989; 37:265-271.

Van Winkle LJ. *Biomembrane Transport.* San Diego, CA: Academic Press, 1995.

Yu-Ling X. Indications of the application of electrochemical therapy. In: *Proceedings of the Fourth International Symposium on Biologically Closed Electric Circuits*. Bloomington, MN: International Association for Biologically Closed Electric Circuits in Biomedicine, pgs 52-58, October 26-29, 1997.

Yuan J, Glazer PM. Mutagenesis induced by the tumor microenvironment. *Mutat Res* 1998; 400:439–446.

Yuan J, Narayanan L, Rockwell S, Glazer PM. Diminished DNA repair and elevated mutagenesis in mammalian cells exposed to hypoxia and low pH. *Cancer Res* 2000; 60:4372–4376.

Chapter V

Classical Description of Tumor Life: Boltzamann Equation for Cancer Tumor Evolution

Introduction

Since 2002, cancer has become the leading cause of death for Americans between the ages of 40 and 74 (Jemal, 2005). But the overall effectiveness of therapeutic cancer treatments is only 50%. Understanding tumor biology and developing an effective prognostic tool could, therefore, have immediate impact on the lives of millions of people diagnosed with cancer. There is growing recognition that achieving an integrative understanding of molecules, cells, tissues, and organs is the next major frontier of biomedical science. Because of the inherent complexity of real biological systems, the development and analysis of computational models based directly on experimental data is necessary to achieve this understanding.

Tumor development is very complex and dynamic. Primary malignant tumors arise from small nodes of cells that have lost, or ceased to respond to, normal growth-regulating mechanisms, through mutations and/or altered gene expression (Sutherland, 1988). This genetic instability causes continued malignant alterations, resulting in a biologically complex tumor. However, all tumors start from a relatively simpler, avascular stage of growth, with nutrient supply by diffusion from the surrounding tissue. The restricted supply of critical nutrients, such as oxygen and glucose, results in marked gradients within the cell mass. The tumor cells respond both through induced alterations in physiology and metabolism, and through altered gene and protein expression (Marusic, 1994), leading to the secretion of a wide variety of angiogenic factors.

Angiogenesis – formation of new blood vessels from existing blood vessels – is necessary for subsequent tumor expansion. Angiogenic growth factors generated by tumor cells diffuse into the nearby tissues and bind to specific receptors on the endothelial cells of nearby pre-existing blood vessels. The endothelial cells become activated, after which they proliferate and migrate towards the tumor, generating blood vessel tubes that connect to form blood vessel loops that can circulate blood. With the new supply system, the tumor will renew growth at a much faster rate. Cells can invade the surrounding tissues and use their new blood supply as highways to travel to other parts of the body. Members of the vascular endothelial growth factor (VEGF) family are known to have a predominant role in angiogenesis.

Physicists have long been at the forefront of cancer diagnosis and treatment, having pioneered the use of X-rays and radiation therapy. In the contemporary initiative, the US National Cancer Institute's conviction that physicists bring unique conceptual insights that could augment the more traditional approaches to cancer research is very appealing.

In this chapter, we present the first attempt to consider the tumor cancer as a physical medium with some sort of memory.

The Consciousness of Cancer Cells

Cancer is pervasive among all organisms in which adult cells proliferate. There is a Darwinian explanation of cancer insidiousness which is based on the fact that all life on Earth was originally single-celled. Each cell had a basic imperative: replicate, replicate, replicate. However, the emergence of multicellular organisms about 550 million years ago required individual cells to co-operate by subordinating their own selfish genetic agenda to that of the organism as a whole. So when an embryo develops, identical stern cells progressively-differentiate into specialized cells that differ from organ to organ.

If a cell does not respond properly to the regulatory signals of the organism, it may continue reproducing in an uncontrolled way, forming a tumor specific to the organ in which it arises. A key hallmark of cancer is that it can also grow in an organ where it does not belong: for example, a prostate cancer cell may grow in a lymph mode. This spreading and invasion processes is called "metastasis." Metastatic cells may lie dormant for many years in foreign organs, evading the body's immune system while retaining their potency. Healthy cells, in contrast, soon die if they are transported beyond their rightful organ.

In some respect, the self-centered nature of cancer cells is a reversion to an ancient pre-multicellular lifestyle. Nevertheless, cancer cells do co-operate to a certain extent. For example, tumors create their own new bloody supply, a phenomenon called "angiogenesis," by co-opting the body's normal wound-healing functions. Cancer cells are therefore neither rogue "selfish cells" nor do they display the collective discipline of an organism with fully-differentiated organs. They fall somewhere in between, perhaps resembling an early form of loosely-organized cell colonies. In other words, the cancer tumor remembers the early state of existence – it has a memory which has been erased in healthy cells.

The proliferation of the tumor cells is described by the diffusion processes (Jamal, 2005). The standard diffusion equation is based on the Fourier law in which, as we know, all memory of the initial state is erased. Simply speaking, the diffusion equation does not have time reversal symmetry, i.e. if the function $f(x, t)$ is the solution of Fourier equation, $f(x, -t)$ is not.

Let us consider the one-dimensional transport "particles", e.g. cancer cells. These cells, however, may move only to the right or to the left. Moving cells may interact with the fixed host body cells, the probabilities of such collisions and their expected results being specified.

All particles will be of the same kind, with the same energy and other physical specifications distinguishable only by their direction.

Let us define:

$u(z, t)$ = expected density of cells at z and at time t moving to the right,

$v(z, t)$ = expected density of cells at z and at time t moving to the left.

Furthermore, let

$\delta(z)$ = probability of collision occurring between a fixed scattering centrum and a cell moving between z and $z+\Delta$.

Suppose that a collision might result in the disappearance of the moving cell without new particle appearing. Such a phenomenon is called *absorption*. Or the moving particle may be reversed in direction or back-scattered. We shall agree that in each collision at z, an expected total of $F(z)$ cells arises moving in the direction of the original cell, while $B(z)$ arise going in the opposite direction.

The expected total number of right-moving cells $z_1 \le z \le z_2$ at time t is

$$\int_{z_1}^{z_2} u(z,t)dz \quad , \tag{1}$$

while the total number of cell passing z to the right in the time interval $t_1 \le t \le t_2$ is

$$w\int_{t_1}^{t_2} u(z,t)dt \quad , \tag{2}$$

where w is the particles speed.

Consider the cell moving to the right and passing $z+\Delta$ in the time interval $t_1 + \frac{\Delta}{w} \le t \le t_2 + \frac{\Delta}{w}$:

$$w\int_{t_1+\Delta/w}^{t_2+\Delta/w} u(z+\Delta,t')dt' = w\int_{t_1}^{t_2} u\left(z+\Delta, t'+\frac{\Delta}{w}\right)dt'. \tag{3}$$

These can arise from cells which passed z in the time interval $t_1 \le t \le t_2$ and came through $(z, z+\Delta)$ without collision

$$w\int_{t_1}^{t_2} (1-\Delta\delta(z,t'))u(z,t')dt' \tag{4}$$

in addition to contributions from collisions in the interval ($z, z+\Delta$). The right-moving cells interacting in ($z, z+\Delta$) produce in the time t_1 to t_2,

$$w\int_{t_1}^{t_2} \Delta\delta(z,t')F(z,t')u(z,t')dt' \tag{5}$$

cells to the right, while the left moving ones give:

$$w\int_{t_1}^{t_2} \Delta\delta(z,t')B(z,t')v(z,t')dt' \quad . \tag{6}$$

Thus,

$$w\int_{t_1}^{t_2} u\left(z+\Delta, t'+\frac{\Delta}{w}\right)dt' = w\int_{t_1}^{t_2} u(z,t')dt' + w\Delta\int_{t_1}^{t_2} \delta(z,t')(F(z,t')-1)u(z,t')dt'$$
$$+w\Delta\int_{t_1}^{t_2} \delta(z,t')B(z,t')v(z,t')dt'. \tag{7}$$

Now, we can write:

$$u\left(z+\Delta, t'+\frac{\Delta}{w}\right) = u(z,t') + \left(\frac{\partial u}{\partial z}(z,t') + \frac{1}{w}\frac{\partial u}{\partial t}(z,t')\right)\Delta \tag{8}$$

to get

$$\int_{t_1}^{t_2} \left(\frac{\partial u}{\partial z}(z,t')\right) + \frac{1}{w}\frac{\partial u}{\partial t}(z,t')dt' = \int_{t_1}^{t_2} \delta(z,t')((F(z,t')-1)u(z,t') + B(z,t')v(z,t'))dt'. \tag{9}$$

On letting $\Delta \to 0$ and differentiating with respect to t_2 we find

$$\frac{\partial u}{\partial z} + \frac{1}{w}\frac{\partial u}{\partial t} = \delta(z,t)(F(z,t)-1)u(z,t) + \delta(z,t)B(z,t)v(z,t). \tag{10}$$

In a like manner,

$$-\frac{\partial v}{\partial z}+\frac{1}{w}\frac{\partial v}{\partial t}=\delta(z,t)B(z,t)u(z,t)+\delta(z,t)(F(z,t)-1)v(z,t). \tag{11}$$

The system of partial differential equations of hyperbolic type (10,11) is the Boltzmann equation for one dimensional transport phenomena (Kozlowski, Marciak-Kozlowska, 2009). Let us define the total density for cells, $\rho(z,t)$

$$\rho(z,t)=u(z,t)+v(z,t) \tag{12}$$

and density of cells current

$$j(z,t)=w(u(z,t)-v(z,t)). \tag{13}$$

Considering equations (12,13), one obtains

$$\frac{\partial \rho}{\partial z}+\frac{1}{w^2}\frac{\partial j}{\partial t}=\delta(z,t)u(z,t)(F(z,t)-B(z,t)-1)+\delta(z,t)v(z,t)(B(z,t)-F(z,t)+1). \tag{14}$$

Equation (14) can be written as

$$\frac{\partial \rho}{\partial z}+\frac{1}{w^2}\frac{\partial j}{\partial t}=\frac{\delta(z,t)(F(z,t)-B(z,t)-1)j}{w} \tag{15}$$

or

$$j=\frac{w}{\delta(z,t)(F(z,t)-B(z,t)-1)}\frac{\partial \rho}{\partial z}+\frac{1}{w\delta(z,t)(F(z,t)-B(z,t)-1)}\frac{\partial j}{\partial t}. \tag{16}$$

Denoting D, diffusion coefficient

$$D=-\frac{w}{\delta(z,t)(F(z,t)-B(z,t)-1)}$$

and τ, relaxation time

$$\tau=\frac{1}{w\delta(z,t)(1-F(z,t)-B(z,t))} \tag{17}$$

Equation (16) takes the form

$$j = -D\frac{\partial \rho}{\partial z} - \tau\frac{\partial j}{\partial t}. \tag{18}$$

Equation (18) is the Cattaneo's type equation and is the generalization of the Fourier equation (Kozlowski, Marciak-Kozlowska, 2009). Now, in a like manner, we obtain from equation (15,18)

$$\frac{1}{w}\frac{\partial j}{\partial z} + \frac{1}{w}\frac{\partial \rho}{\partial t} = \delta(z,t)u(z,t)(F(z,t) - 1 + B(z,t))$$
$$+\delta(z,t)v(z,t)(B(z,t) + F(z,t) - 1)) \tag{19}$$

or

$$\frac{\partial j}{\partial z} + \frac{\partial \rho}{\partial t} = 0. \tag{20}$$

Equation (20) describes the conservation of cells in the transport processes.

Considering equations (19) and (20) for the constant D and τ, the hyperbolic Heaviside equation is obtained:

$$\tau\frac{\partial^2 \rho}{\partial t^2} + \frac{\partial \rho}{\partial t} = D\frac{\partial^2 \rho}{\partial z^2}. \tag{21}$$

where τ is the relaxation time.

In the stationary state, transport phenomena $dF(z,t)/dt = dB(z,t)dt = 0$ and $d\delta(z,t)/dt = 0$. In that case, we denote $F(z,t) = F(z) = B(z,t) = B(z) = k(z)$ and equation (10) and (11) can be written as

$$\frac{du}{dz} = \delta(z)(k-1)u(z) + \delta(z)kv(z),$$
$$-\frac{dv}{dz} = \delta(z)k(z)u(z) + \delta(z)(k(z)-1)v(z) \tag{22}$$

with diffusion coefficient

$$D = \frac{w}{\delta(z)} \tag{23}$$

and relaxation time

$$\tau(z) = \frac{1}{w\delta(z)(1-2k(z))}. \tag{24}$$

The system of equations (22) can be written as

$$\frac{d^2u}{dz^2} - \frac{\frac{d}{dz}(\delta k)}{\delta k}\frac{du}{dz} + u\left[\delta^2(2k-1) + \frac{d\delta}{dz}(1-k) + \frac{\delta(k-1)}{\delta k}\frac{d(\delta k)}{dz}\right] = 0, \tag{25}$$

$$\frac{du}{dz} = \delta(k-1)u + \delta k v(z). \tag{26}$$

Equation (25) after differentiation has the form

$$\frac{d^2u}{dz^2} + f(z)\frac{du}{dz} + g(z)u(z) = 0, \tag{27}$$

where

$$f(z) = -\frac{1}{\delta}\left(\frac{\delta}{k}\frac{dk}{dz} + \frac{d\delta}{dz}\right),$$
$$g(z) = \delta^2(z)(2k-1) - \frac{\delta}{k}\frac{dk}{dz}. \tag{28}$$

For the constant absorption rate we put

$$k(z) = k = \text{constant} \neq \frac{1}{2}.$$

In that case,

$$f(z) = -\frac{1}{\delta}\frac{d\delta}{dz},$$
$$g(z) = \delta^2(z)(zk-1). \tag{29}$$

With functions $f(z)$ and $g(z)$, the general solution of the equation (27) has the form

$$u(z) = C_1 e^{(1-2k)^{1/2}\int \delta dz} + C_2 e^{-(1-2k)^{1/2}\int \delta dz} \tag{30}$$

Subsequently, we will consider the solution of the equation (2.32) with $f(z)$ and $g(z)$ described by (2.34) for Cauchy condition:

$$u(0) = q, \quad v(a) = 0 \tag{31}$$

Boundary condition (27) describes the generation of the heat carriers (by illuminating the left end of the strand with laser pulses) with velocity q heat carrier per second.

The solution has the form:

$$u(z) = \frac{2qe^{[f(0)-f(a)]}}{1+\beta e^{2[f(0)-f(a)]}}\left[\frac{(1-2k)^{\frac{1}{2}}}{(1-2k)^{\frac{1}{2}}-(k-1)}\right]\cosh[f(x)-f(a)]$$

$$+\frac{k-1}{(1-2k)^{\frac{1}{2}}-(k-1)}\sinh[f(x)-f(a)],$$

$$u(z) = \frac{2qe^{(f(0)-f(a))}}{1+\beta e^{2[f(0)-f(a)]}}\left[\frac{(1-2k)^{\frac{1}{2}}+(k-1)}{k}\sinh[f(x)-f(a)]\right], \tag{32}$$

where

$$f(z) = (1-2k)^{\frac{1}{2}}\int \delta dz,$$

$$f(0) = (1-2k)^{\frac{1}{2}}\left[\int \delta dz\right]_0,$$

$$f(a) = (1-2k)^{\frac{1}{2}}\left[\int \delta dz\right]_a,$$

$$\beta = \frac{(1-2k)^{\frac{1}{2}}+(k-1)}{(1-2k)^{\frac{1}{2}}-(k-1)}. \tag{33}$$

Considering formulae (31,32), we obtain for the density $\rho(z)$ and current density $j(z)$.

$$j(z) = \frac{2qwe^{[f(0)-f(a)]}}{1+\beta e^{2[f(0)-f(a)]}} \left[\begin{array}{l} \dfrac{(1-2k)^{\frac{1}{2}}}{(1-2k)^{\frac{1}{2}} - (k-1)} \cosh[f(z) - f(a)] \\ - \dfrac{1-2k}{(1-2k)^{\frac{1}{2}} - (k-1)} \sinh[f(z) - f(a)] \end{array} \right] \tag{34}$$

and

$$q = \frac{2qe^{[f(0)-f(a)]}}{1+\beta e^{2[f(0)-f(a)]}} \left[\begin{array}{l} \dfrac{(1-2k)^{\frac{1}{2}}}{(1-2k)^{\frac{1}{2}} - (k-1)} \cosh[f(z) - f(a)] \\ - \dfrac{1}{(1-2k)^{\frac{1}{2}} - (k-1)} \sinh[f(z) - f(a)] \end{array} \right]. \tag{35}$$

Equations (34) and (35) fulfill the generalized Fourier relation

$$j = -\frac{w}{\delta(z)} \frac{\partial \rho}{\partial z}, \qquad D = \frac{W}{\delta(z)}, \tag{36}$$

where D denotes the diffusion coefficient.

Analogously, we define the generalized diffusion velocity $\upsilon_D(z)$

$$\upsilon_D(z) = \frac{j(z)}{n(z)} = \frac{w(1-2k)^{\frac{1}{2}} \left[\cosh[f(z) - f(a)] - (1-2k)^{\frac{1}{2}} \sinh[f(x) - f(a)] \right]}{(1-2k)^{\frac{1}{2}} \cosh[f(x) - f(a)] - \sinh[f(x) - f(a)]}. \tag{37}$$

Assuming constant cross section for heat carriers scattering $\delta(z) = \delta_o$ we obtain from formula (36)

$$\begin{aligned} &f(z) = (1-2k)^{\frac{1}{2}} z, \\ &f(0) = 0, \\ &f(a) = (1-2k)^{\frac{1}{2}} a \end{aligned} \tag{38}$$

and for density $\rho(z)$ and current density $j(z)$

$$j(z)=\frac{2qwe^{-(1-2k)^{\frac{1}{2}}a\delta}}{1+\beta e^{-(1-2k)^{\frac{1}{2}}a\delta}}\left[\frac{(1-2k)^{\frac{1}{2}}}{(1-2k)^{\frac{1}{2}}-(k-1)}\cosh\left[(2k-1)^{\frac{1}{2}}(x-a)\delta\right]\right.$$
$$\left.-\frac{(1-2k)}{(1-2k)^{\frac{1}{2}}-(k-1)}\sinh\left[(2k-1)^{\frac{1}{2}}(x-a)\delta\right]\right], \tag{39}$$

$$\rho(z)=\frac{2qe^{-(1-2k)^{\frac{1}{2}}a\delta}}{1+\beta e^{-(1-2k)^{\frac{1}{2}}a\delta}}\left[\frac{(1-2k)^{\frac{1}{2}}}{(1-2k)^{\frac{1}{2}}-(k-1)}\cosh\left[(2k-1)^{\frac{1}{2}\delta}(x-a)\right]\right.$$
$$\left.-\frac{1}{(1-2k)^{\frac{1}{2}}-(k-1)}\sinh\left[(2k-1)^{\frac{1}{2}}(x-a)\delta\right]\right]. \tag{40}$$

Formulae (39) and (40) describe the kinetic of the growth of the cell aggregation-tumor. The development of the tumor strongly depends on the coefficient *k*. In the following, we will call *k* the growth coefficient. For $k<0.5$ the density of the cell oscillate, Figure 1a, 2a. On the other hand for $k>0.5$ the cell density grows exponentially, Figure 2a, 2b.

For $k<0.5$ the cell aggregation emits the wave with length λ=size of the tumor. For $k=0.5$ the cancer development has a cusp, Figure 1a. For k=1.91 density of the tumor cells has a singularity. For $k<0.5$ the density of the cell oscillate, Figure 2a. On the other hand, for $k>0.5$ the cell density grows exponentially, Figure 2b.

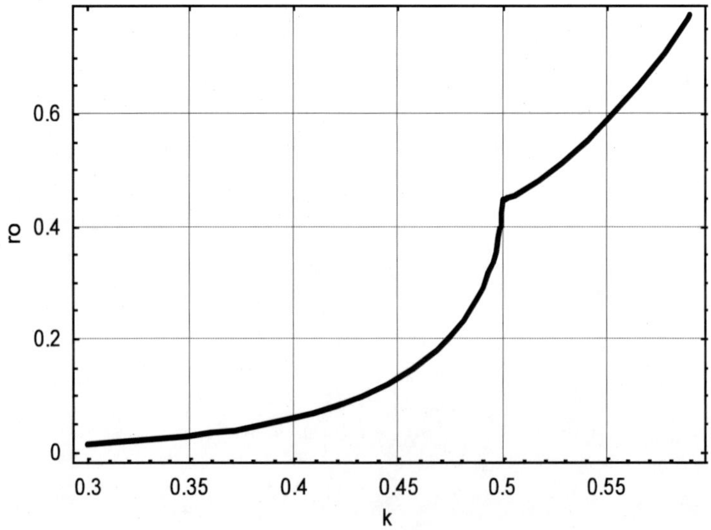

Figure 1a. Cells density, formula (2.45) as the function of the growth factor k, for x=3 um, a=1 um.

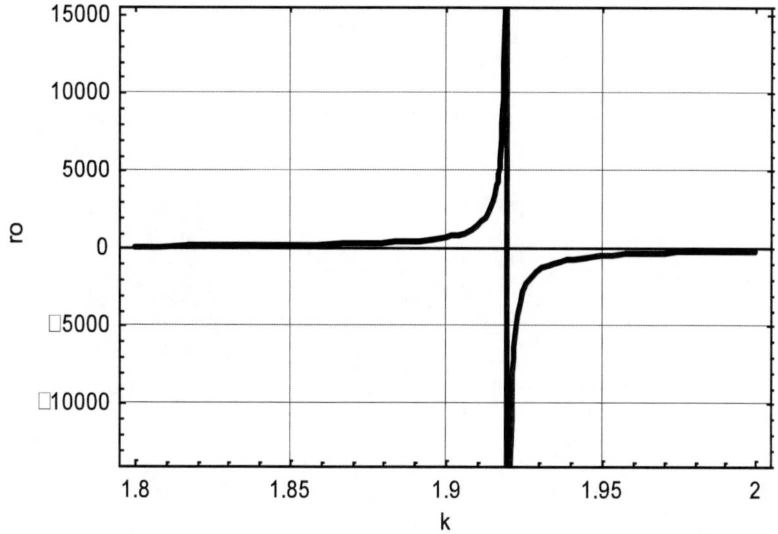

Figure 1b. The same as in Figure 1a, but for k>0.5

We will call the first stage *k<0.5* the "hesitation" period in which a tumor sends the "information" waves to the host body. The response of the host depends on its willingness to cooperate with cancer. *For k<0.5* the response of the host is *negative* and the tumor is stable. For *k>0.5* the *angiogenesis* starts – the host cooperates with the tumor and the tumor grows abruptly.

It seems that the first "hesitation" stage is the exchange of the information from tumor→ host→ tumor and *vice versa*. Next, through the singularity point *k=1.9, for x=3 um* the cancer obtains the information "*go*" and *metastasis* process starts.

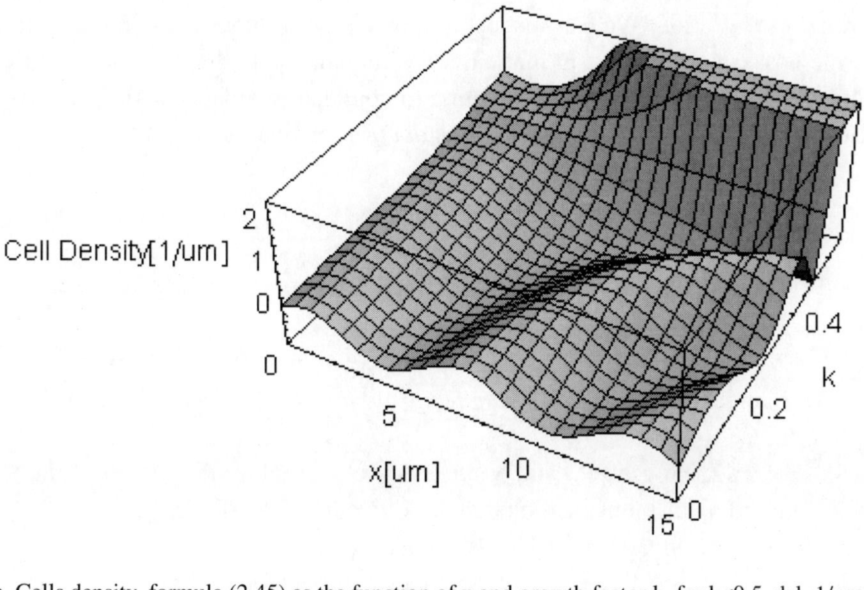

Figure 2a. Cells density, formula (2.45) as the function of x and growth factor k, for k<0.5, del=1/um, a=10 um.

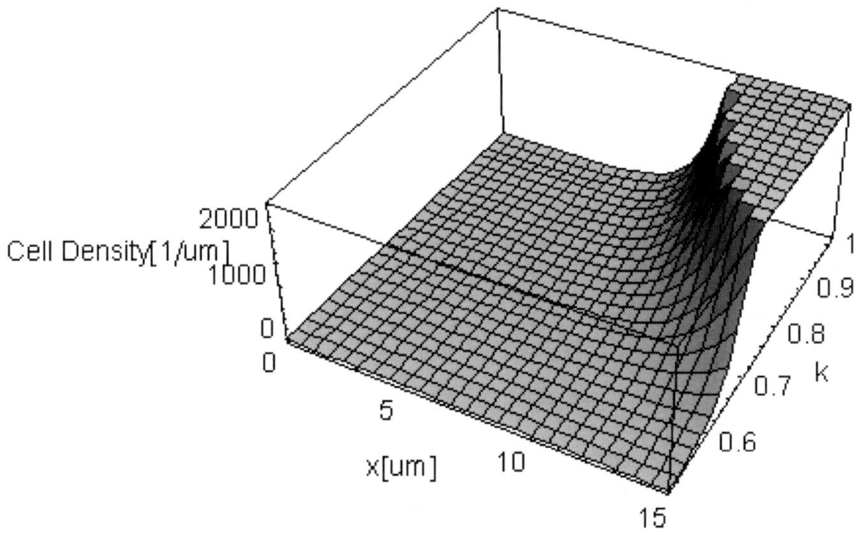

Figure 2b. The same as in Figure 2a, but for k>0.5, del=1/um,

From the therapeutic point of view, the most important result of the paper is the description of the "information-conscious" waves in the host body.

In this paragraph, we argue that the cancer tumor evolution can be described as the process which strongly depends on the growth factor *k*, defined in the chapter. For *k*<0.5 the tumor is stable with oscillatory behavior of the cells density. For *k*> 0.5 the tumor grows exponentially. For the moment, the tumor wave emission was not observed. It seems that the observation of the emitted waves can be an important therapeutic tool for the description of the cancer status. The stop of the emission of the waves is the signature of the invasive evolution of the tumor. It seems that the host is informed by emitted waves on the existence of the tumor and its evolution. We can suspect the same sort of tumor consciousness which can influence the host consciousness. In that case, we can anticipate the correlation of the tumor growth and psychic of the host. It is interesting to note that in a paper by Erica K. Sloan and others (Sloan, 2010), the role of the *neuroendoctrine* activation in cancer propagation is described and investigated.

References

Jemal, A.: *The Journal of the American Medical Association*, 200; 294:1255–1259.

Kozlowski M. Marciak-Kozlowska J. *From femto- to attoscience and beyond*, NOVA, USA, 2009

Marusic, M., Bajzer Z, Freyer J.P., and Vuk-Pavlovic S: Analysis of growth of multicellular tumour spheroid by mathematical models. *Cell Prolif.* 1994; 27; 73 -78

Sloan Erica, K, et. al., *Cancer Res*, 2010; 70 (18) 7042-7052

Sutherland, R.M. Cell and environment interactions in tumor microregions: the multicell spheroid model. *Science*, 1988; 240:177–184.

Chapter VI

Quantum Mechanics and Cancer

Introduction

Quantum mechanics is a highly successful theory which accurately describes physical reality in a wide range of situations. Its use of the non-intuitive wave function, however, means that the true nature of the physical reality described is far from clear. Because of this, many different interpretations—conceptual pictures of the nature of the underlying reality—have been proposed. There are three major interpretations and perhaps a dozen others, so one sometimes gets the impression that it is not possible to gain a proper understanding of what underlies the theory.

The situation, however, is not as chaotic as it appears. The reason there are so many interpretations is that their originators were apparently not aware of *all* the relevant properties of the theory itself. So what we do here is list and justify all the properties of quantum mechanics relevant to its interpretation. This approach brings order to the interpretive problem and significantly narrows down the set of possible interpretations.

History. To understand how a successful theory could require an interpretation, we need to briefly review the history of physics. Classical mechanics, discovered almost entirely by Newton around 1700, was a very successful mathematical scheme for predicting the paths of the atoms of which matter was presumably constituted. Since it involved the flight of easily-visualized particles through our familiar three-dimensional space, classical physics gave a picture of reality which was compatible with our conventional, everyday view of the world. Quantum mechanics, however, is a different story. It was discovered in the search for a mathematical scheme which would explain classically-unsolvable problems, such as the spectrum of electromagnetic radiation given off by a hot object, the photoelectric effect, and especially why the hydrogen atom radiates certain colors of light. Rather than being the brainchild of a single person, however, there were at least half a dozen major physicists who, over a period of 25 years, each discovered an essential piece of the puzzle. And with each piece, the mathematics moved farther away from our everyday view of the world.

The end result of these separate insights—the equation discovered by Schrödinger in 1926—was a scheme which is highly successful. In addition to the hydrogen atom spectrum, quantum mechanics describes a great many phenomena—all the properties of atoms and nuclei, semiconductors, lasers, the systematics of elementary particles—and it has never given a result in conflict with experiment. But its mathematics involves the mysterious wave function rather than the easily-visualized particles, so it no longer has a clear correspondence with our commonplace view of reality. Because of this, one needs an *interpretation* of the mathematics to understand how it relates to our perceived physical world.

Peculiarities of Quantum Mechanics

Quantum mechanics is difficult to understand because it has two peculiar properties. The first, illustrated by the Schrödinger's cat experiment in the next section, is that the wave function contains several *simultaneously existing* versions of reality—the cat is both alive and dead at the same time. We perceive only one of those possible versions of reality. But quantum mechanics treats all versions equally, so it does not tell us why we perceive a *particular* version.

The fact that there are several versions of reality leads to the second peculiar property – probability. Through an empirically verified law which currently *appears* to be separate from the rest of the mathematics, quantum mechanics tells us the *probability* of seeing a live cat or a dead cat. There is currently no clear understanding of this 'rolling-the-dice' aspect of the theory. (There is one other peculiar quantum mechanical property, non-locality—see appendix A6. But, although it is of interest in its own right, non-locality is not a major factor in determining the correct interpretation.)

*Major interpretations***.** There are three major interpretations which attempt to give an understanding of these properties. The first is to suppose that, in addition to the many quantum versions of reality, there is an actual, objective reality made of particles, and it is the particles, rather than the wave functions, that we perceive. A second potential way out of the multiple-versions-of-reality problem is to suppose the wave function 'collapses' down to just one version. The dead cat wave function might collapse to zero, for example, leaving just a live cat (wave function) to be perceived. And a third possible solution, the Everett many-worlds interpretation, is to suppose all versions always exist, so there are many version of each of us! We will explain these in more detail and show that each—including the existence of particles!—runs into severe difficulties.

Mathematics and perceptions. We perceive a world that has only a single version of reality and so we naturally assume that the 'actual' reality consists of only a single, 'objective' version of reality. Further, because the classical physics of Newton worked so well, we tend to assume that the world is made up of particles. But this 'intuitively obvious' scheme—a single-version reality made up of particles—is not our starting point. What we are most certain of are (1) our perceptions and (2) the mathematics which describes what we perceive so well. So, in the quest to deduce the true nature of the physical world from physics, we use the strategy of examining the connections between the *mathematics* of quantum mechanics and our *perceptions.* In this way, we hope to eliminate any prejudgments on the nature of reality. This approach, as we will see, leads us in unexpected directions. It is not possible to adequately explain the basic ideas without a firm grasp of the interpretations of quantum mechanics. Thus, this chapter is organized around interpretations. Our treatment of them will appear to be unorthodox to some. But to the best of our knowledge, *all* the relevant principles of quantum mechanics are taken into account here and/or in [1], in a carefully organized way, and that is not true of most other inquiries into interpretations.

Visualizing the wave function. The Schrödinger equation of quantum mechanics governs the motion of the *wave functions*, so it is (on the least abstract level) the wave functions which are the 'physical objects' in the mathematics of quantum mechanics; particles never enter the mathematics. A useful visual picture of the wave function is that it is matter spread out in a mist or cloud of varying density. The Schrödinger equation determines the shape and density of the cloud, and how it moves through space. If there are several 'particles,' the total wave function may be pictured as several separate (or sometimes overlapping) clouds, with the Schrödinger equation determining how the clouds interact. The wave function of a macroscopic object like a cat or a human being, composed of billions of 'single particle' individual wave functions, is extremely complicated, but that does not prevent us from deducing certain relevant general characteristics.

Many versions of reality. The world around us certainly appears to be *the* unique physical world upon which we all agree. But in quantum mechanics, the highly-successful mathematical description of nature, there is no unique physical world; instead, there are many simultaneously-existing *versions* of physical reality. We will give two examples here: nuclear decay and Schrödinger's cat. Two other examples of simultaneously existing versions of reality, involving the polarization of light and the spin of particles, are given in appendices A1 and A2. These two phenomena are important because they are often used in theoretical arguments, both here and in the general literature, and in the experiments employed to test the peculiarities of quantum mechanics.

Schrödinger's cat. The Schrödinger's cat experiment (1935) is a clever and dramatic way of boosting this strange multi-reality situation from the atomic (nuclear) to the macroscopic level. A cat is put in a box along with a vial of cyanide. Outside the box are a radioactive source and a detector of the radiation. The detector is turned on for five seconds and then turned off. If it records one or more counts of radiation, an electrical signal is sent to the box, the vial of cyanide is broken, and the cat dies. If it records no counts, nothing happens and the cat lives.

Classically, there is no problem here (unless you are a cat lover). Either the nucleus radioactively decays, the cat dies, and you perceive a dead cat when you open the box; or the nucleus does not decay, the cat lives, and you perceive a live cat. Schematically, in the classical case,

either

[cat dies] [you perceive a dead cat]

or

[cat lives] [you perceive a live cat]

But this is not what happens in the quantum case. There, the wave function of the nucleus, the cat, and you (as the observer) is

[cat dies]
[version 1: you perceives a dead cat]
and, simultaneously
[cat lives]
[version 2: you perceives a live cat]

There are now two full-blown, simultaneously-existing versions of physical reality. In one, there is a dead version of the cat, in the other there is a live version. In version 1, you perceive a dead cat, in the other, version 2, you perceive a live cat. So in quantum mechanics, there are *two simultaneously existing, equally valid versions of you*, each perceiving something different!

In reality, your perceptions will correspond to one version or the other (but that does not necessarily imply that only one version 'exists').

Agreement of quantum mechanics with our perceptions. Schrödinger's cat gives an illustration of a set of general properties which follow from the agreement in all known cases between observation and the quantum mechanically-predicted characteristics of the versions of reality:

1. Quantum mechanics gives many *potential* versions of reality.
2. In all instances where the calculations and observations can be done, there is always one and only one version whose characteristics corresponds exactly—qualitatively and quantitatively—to our physical perceptions.
3. Quantum mechanics does not single out any version for perception.
4. All observers agree on the perceived version.
5. Each version of reality corresponds to a different, isolated universe. There can be no communication of any kind—via light, sound, touch, email, and so on—between the different versions.

Classical consistency of observation (See appendix A3 for details). The tendency is to suppose that, because quantum mechanics contains several simultaneously existing versions of reality, it must be that in the un-amended theory (no collapse), we should *perceive* several simultaneous versions of reality, akin to a double exposure. But that is not correct. In quantum mechanics proper (the QMA of section 4), *the observer perceives only one version.* Each version, however, is in a separate, isolated universe and can therefore perceive only what is in that universe; a version in one universe can never perceive what occurs in a separate universe. And there is nothing in QMA that perceives in more than one universe. Thus,

6. Perception of more than one outcome of an experiment can never occur within quantum mechanics. If we look in the box twice after doing the Schrödinger's cat experiment, we certainly expect, from experience, to see the same thing both times. One can show that this holds in quantum mechanics also.
7. If two observations are made successively, quantum mechanics implies the same consistency of results as one obtains in a classical universe.

8. A technical version of 7 is that if one *measures* the same property twice in a row, quantum mechanics implies one will get the same result.

Finally, in addition to an observer perceiving only one version of reality, we also know experientially that two observers never disagree on what they perceive. But this also follows from quantum mechanics.

9. Quantum mechanics implies that two observers can never disagree on what they perceive.

Principles 5 through 9 constitute much of the content of what is called measurement theory. (There is also a principle about perceiving only the eigenvalues of relevant operators, but that is not relevant here.) They show that in all circumstances, quantum mechanics itself implies a 'classical' consistency of perceptual results even though no classical (that is, single-version-of-reality, effect-follows-from-cause) reality was assumed.

Quantum physics and biology. Quantum physics includes a wide variety of phenomena. Most of them are regarded as unusual because they violate our everyday expectations of how nature should behave.

Quantum physics derives its very name from the discreteness of nature. The Latin word 'quantum' is used to ask the question 'how much?' and even colloquially, a quantum is nowadays a small portion. Several physical properties only assume a countable number of values. This is, for instance, true for the electronic energy in atoms or the vibrational energy in molecules. The quantized set of spectral lines, Figure 1a, is often used in the life sciences as a finger print of chemical substances, since it relates to the discrete set of energies in all nanomatter, from atoms to large biomolecules. And yet, this aspect is regarded as atomic and chemical physics rather than a part of quantum biology. If, however, single photons or single spins can trigger a chain of macroscopic phenomena in organic systems, the assignment will be justified.

One of the intriguing aspects of physics is related to the fact that quantum states are well-defined even when they refer to situations which we would describe as a coexistence of mutually-excluding possibilities in classical physics. We usually adhere to Aristotle's principle of non-contradiction, that the same attribute cannot at the same time belong and not belong to the same subject. Quantum physics teaches us that we either have to give up this wisdom or otherwise renounce other well-established intellectual concepts, such as our understanding of reality, information, or space-time. A paradigmatic example for this fact is the dual nature of light, which manifests itself in Young's famous double-slit diffraction experiment (Figure 1b). When a light beam is sent onto a small opening in a wall, it will spread out behind the slit. If we open a neighboring slit in the screen, we will observe a fringe pattern (Figure 1b) that exhibits dark minima at several screen positions that are still bright when only a single slit is open. This observation is explained by the superposition and interference of classical electromagnetic waves of well-defined relative phases, i.e. sufficient mutual coherence. The same wave interference experiment turns into a quantum puzzle when we dilute the optical field to the level of individual quanta of light, photons, which are always detected as localized packets of energy, $E = h\nu$. The delocalized nature of photons in free flight and their localized character in the detection process is at the heart of their wave-particle duality and very incompatible with classical reasoning. Here, ν relates the frequency of the electromagnetic wave to the energy E of each individual photon through Planck's constant of action h. The superposition principle is also associated with the dualism between determinism and quantum randomness: the shape and location of the envelope of the interference pattern is strictly determined by a wave equation. The square of the wave amplitude represents the probability to detect a single event. Each individual realization is, however, objectively random within the predetermined probabilities. Quantum theory describes the evolution of delocalized objects perfectly well, but a measurement signifies a break in this evolution and introduces a random element. Since it terminates the wave-like propagation of the quantum state, it is often described as a collapse of the wave function. It is still an open debate whether measurements have an ontological or, rather, an epistemological meaning, i.e. whether they describe an outside reality or our knowledge about the world. But for many practical purposes, the act of measurement is a valid and useful concept. It is important to note that interference always occurs, when the wave associated to a quantum object may reach the detector along at least two different but intrinsically indistinguishable paths – either in real-space or in some configuration space (e.g. potential curves). The Mach-Zehnder interferometer, sketched in Figure 1d, is a simple textbook arrangement, which is often used to demonstrate delocalization and interference for photons over macroscopic distances. It also visualizes an idea that has been invoked in the description of coherent energy transport in organic molecules. Diffraction and interference deviate even more from our classical expectations when we observe them with massive particles, such as electrons, neutrons, or atoms (Cronin et al., 2009, and citations therein). But chemistry teaches us that the delocalization of electrons over nanometers is rather ubiquitous, for instance across the bonds of aromatic molecules. The wave-nature of matter is also of relevance for life science in a different context: the short de Broglie wave length of fast electrons allows to obtain high resolution images in electron microscopy and neutron waves are useful in analyzing crystallized protein structures. While electrons and neutrons are still rather small and elementary particles, recent experiments were able to demonstrate the delocalization of entire molecules, such as C60, using far-field diffraction (Arndt et al., 1999). And even biodyes, such as porphyrin derivatives, revealed their quantum wave properties in a near-field interferometer (Hackermüller et al., 2003), and briefly outlined below: the molecular powder was evaporated to form a beam, which was velocity selected to $\Delta v/v \simeq 15$–$20\ \%$. The stream was directed onto a gold grating, i.e. an array of slits (450 nm wide) with a period of 990 nm. The molecules are only nanometers large and their center-of-mass is still localized to within a few picometers inside the oven. But once ejected into the vacuum, the free quantum propagation stretches their coherence function by more than a factor of 10,000, i.e. to 50 nm, before they interact with the first grating. Diffraction within the slits of this grating leads to a further broadening of the molecular coherence function, up to several micrometers before the porphyrins encounters the second grating. The simultaneous and indistinguishable passage of the molecular wave amplitude through several slits leads to quantum interference, which manifests itself as a sinusoidal molecular density pattern at the location of the third grating

These experiments show that large scale coherence of biomolecules is obviously observable. These molecules can be delocalized over many micrometers, thousand times their physical size and million times their de Broglie wavelength, and over time scales of a few milliseconds. But it is also clear that this demonstration required laboratory conditions, i.e. high-vacuum conditions to avoid observing interactions with the environment. It is interesting to note that all porphyrin molecules were heated to 690 Kelvin and thermal excitations could drive internal state changes even during the molecular propagation through the interferometer. The reason for de Broglie interference survives lies in the fact that at this temperature, the internal states still remain effectively decoupled from the center-of-mass motion (Hackermüller et al., 2003). Several groups have formulated serious research proposals that ask to which extent quantum superpositions might still be observable on the mass scale, not only of a single organic molecule, but possibly even of a supermassive cluster or a virus (Clauser, 1997; Reiger et al., 2006; Romero-Isart et al., 2009). Chances are high that the idea behind these proposals can actually be successfully implemented within the next decade.

Quantum tunneling. When a particle encounters a potential barrier that is higher than its kinetic energy, it will not be able to pass by any classical means. Quantum mechanics, however, allows it to tunnel through the barrier (see Figure 1c). In order to understand the relevance of this phenomenon for biology, it is important to see that the tunneling probability depends exponentially on the height, width, and shape of the potential barrier. The particle's mass and kinetic energy enter in a similar way. This explains why tunneling of electrons and protons are rather ubiquitous in biology whereas it is unobserved for entire amino acids or proteins: their mass and their interaction potentials grow with the number of molecular constituents and therefore dramatically decrease the probability for this quantum effect.

Spin: a quantum way to turn around. Angular momentum L is a well-established quantity in classical physics, but quantum physics requires that it appears only with a discrete set of values and orientations. Most particles also possess a spin, i.e. an angular momentum that is not related to any mechanical motion and therefore without any classical analog. Spins may also be brought into superposition of two or more mutually-exclusive states, comparable to a single compass needle pointing both north and south at the same time. In spite of being a pure quantum property, spin is also often responsible for magnetism in biological systems on the molecular level. The spin of protons is also exploited to derive structural and functional properties of organisms (Lauterbur, 1973). Magnetic resonance imaging of human tissue relies on the simultaneous response of many trillion spins in a macroscopic biological volume. It is, however, still an open question whether magnetization in biology can be quantized on a larger scale, whether spin entanglement or mesoscopic coherent spin transport can be found under ambient conditions and with a consequence for biological functionality – a question that is resumed below in the context of the magnetic senses in animals.

Quantum superposition of energy states. If a molecule is excited by a femtosecond optical pulse, the energy-time uncertainty relation $\Delta E \times \Delta t \geq \hbar/2$ ensures that the photon energy is sufficiently undetermined to be resonant with more than a single excited state. Femtosecond spectroscopy has thus become a regular tool for characterizing biomolecular systems (Felker et al., 1982) and the coherent superposition of electronic and vibrational energy states are regularly observed in such experiments. But even when biological systems are exposed to incoherent daylight, excitonic coherences may form between electronically coupled neighboring molecules. In photosynthetic complexes, excitonic coupling across several pigment molecules has been reported (Dahlbom et al., 2001) and coherence in photosynthesis is a major field of current research (see further below).

Quantum statistics. The spin of identical particles also determines their statistical behavior within an ensemble. Bosons – particles with an integer value of the spin quantum number s – tend to occupy the same quantum state when they are prepared to be indistinguishable. Fermions with half-integer quantum numbers, such as electrons, avoid each other under otherwise-identical circumstances. This has important consequences: Pauli's exclusion principle, the stability of matter and the existence of neutron stars are important results for fermions. On the other hand, the existence of lasers and Bose-Einstein condensates are macroscopic effects of boson statistics. The observation of quantum statistics with atoms requires highly-specialized environments, such as μK temperatures and ultra-high vacuum. Interestingly, quantum degeneracy of exciton-polaritons has already been observed in a condensed matter system at T=19 K (Kasprzak et al., 2006). This is much closer to the conditions of life, but at present there is still no experimental evidence for quantum statistics on a macroscopic biological scale. On the other hand, it is worth noting that photons are also bosons with a spin quantum number of s = 1, and non-classical states of light may well be generated in organic systems. Although we don't know of any biological laser, random lasing of artificially dye-infiltrated human tissue has been demonstrated recently (Polson and Vardeny, 2004).

Quantum entanglement and quantum information. When we extend the superposition principle to more than a single object or property, we arrive at the notion of quantum entanglement. By this, we mean a non-classical correlation, an unseparable connection between two objects or properties. Amazingly, once established, this quantum connection may theoretically persist over long distances and times, unless it is perturbed by external interactions and measurements.

The example of polarization-entangled photon-pairs shall illustrate the idea (Figure 1f). When photons are sent onto a properly chosen non-linear crystal, each of them can be converted, with a certain probability, into two photons of lower energy. The polarizations of the two photons is then quantum-correlated, i.e. entangled, in the following sense: none of the two emerging photons has a well-defined polarization before it is measured, but when the two quanta of light are polarization-entangled, we can predict in advance and with certainty that the polarization of both will always be orthogonal to each other. There are several formal definitions and measures of entanglement (Vedral and Plenio, 1998). Generally, the following conditions are required to test for it: first, we have to identify at least two physical subsystems or modes. They must be clearly distinguishable and independently addressable for instance through different frequencies, locations, or detector orientations. Secondly, we have to be able to identify at least two complementary measurements that can be performed on each of these two modes, and it should be possible to gradually vary between the two kinds of measurements. In the photon example, these two criteria are easily fulfilled as the two polarizations are orthogonal and optical elements such as λ/2-plates can transform one into the other. The two twin-photons can be emitted in spatially-separated arms too.

Quantum entanglement has been demonstrated for photons, but also for superconducting circuits, nuclear spins in small molecules, spin noise in atomic ensembles, trapped ions, and other systems (see refs. in Nielsen and Chuang, 2000). All these proof-of-principle demonstration experiments were, again, performed under strictly-controlled environmental conditions, often including ultra-high vacuum and ultra-low temperatures – i.e. conditions that are incompatible with living organisms. Interestingly, entanglement may also be mediated by the exchange of light. And the transmission can be amazingly robust, as shown by the successful quantum teleportation of atomic spin properties from one room temperature atomic ensemble to another, over macroscopic distances through air (Sherson et al., 2006). Electromagnetic radiation might thus be an important coherence mediator, if entanglement should be relevant in life. As of today, several algorithms have been suggested which would actually provide a significant advantage over all classical schemes, when implemented with many qubits (see refs. in Nielsen and Chuang, 2000). Quantum computers are expected to provide faster prime number factoring for crypto-analysis using Shor's algorithm, speed-up in database searches using Grover's algorithm, new insights into quantum games (Eisert et al., 1999), or an exponential speed-up in solving systems of linear equations (Harrow et al., 2009). These developments in quantum information science lead to the question of whether quantum methods may also be relevant for living organisms, which are stunning information-processing devices. Yet, the implementation of quantum circuits in biology, as anywhere else, would require a configuration space that increases exponentially with the number of qubits involved. And given the enormous sensitivity of quantum states to most external perturbations, it is widely believed that the probability of a successful coherent computation will also be exponentially-suppressed under the conditions of life as they are known to us. Until today, first quantum computing circuits and elementary quantum algorithms could be demonstrated using nuclear magnetic resonance (NMR) on a few nuclear spins within an individual biomolecule (Jones et al., 2000, see Figure 3a). These experiments approach a natural setting since they were embedded in a condensed matter environment, even though at only a temperature of a few Kelvin. NMR quantum computing in a dense ensemble is mostly hampered by the difficulty of initializing all molecules to the same ground state, and also the rapid randomization of quantum phases by interactions with the host matrix is a further limiting factor. One may also speculate whether naturally-occurring quantum correlations can be used in biology. Being embedded in a macroscopic system, any initial coherent superposition of a molecule – be it in position, electronic, or vibrational excitations – will rapidly be transformed into entanglement with the environment. One could imagine that this yields a functional benefit. But again, experimental evidence for this and other meaningful quantum information processing in nature still has to be found.

The quantum-to-classical transition. In order to understand the overwhelming success of our classical world-view in the description of biological phenomena we have to understand why quantum effects are usually hard to observe. The kinematic argument is based on the insight that Planck's constant of action h¯ is extremely small. For instance, the de Broglie wavelength λdB = h/mv ≃ 10−35 m of an adult man walking at a speed of 1 m/s is way too small to ever be observed. Here, it is rather the value of the fundamental constants than the intrinsic structure of quantum mechanics which forbid the observation of macroscopic quantum delocalization. The phase-averaging argument adds the insight that quantum interference relies on phase coherence. But small wavelengths are easily dephased in changing environments. Fluctuations of the geometry, electromagnetic fields, or chemical environments will easily alter the conditions for constructive and destructive interference. In most cases, thermal fluctuations will render interference phenomena unobservable when we look at macroscopic molecular ensembles. In fact, this does not necessarily mean that quantum mechanics does not play a role in biology: the stochastic dephasing of destructive quantum interference has recently been even invoked as being responsible for the fast energy transport in the photosynthetic complex (Caruso et al., 2009), as further described below. In contrast to the notion of phase-averaging, we here reserve the term decoherence for processes which actually exchange information between the quantum system and its environment (Zurek, 1991; Joos et al., 2003). Decoherence is closely related to the act of measurement. By definition, a quantum measurement extracts information about a quantum system and correlates it to the pointer of a macroscopic meter. But in contrast to the prescriptions of unitary quantum physics, we never see any macroscopic meter pointing up and down at the same time. A valid explanation for that is given by decoherence theory (Joos and Zeh, 1985): the act of measurement on a quantum superposition state will create entanglement between the system and the meter. The quantumness of the original system is thus diluted to a larger composite system (object and meter) and in most cases, the quantumness of the meter diffuses over the entire detector which may contain some 1020-1025 atoms. This is such an incredible amount of particles that we will never be able to retrieve the original quantum coherence from the enlarged system. In contrast to decoherence theory, for which the unitary evolution of quantum physics always persists – even during a measurement – the model of an objective collapse of the quantum wave function assumes that coherences spontaneously disappear in the act of measurement. Spontaneous collapse models assume that this intrinsic loss of coherence is bound to a certain internal complexity and number of participating particles (Ghirardi et al., 1986). Recently, it has also been suggested that the inevitable coupling between mass and deformations of spacetime might cause an objective collapse of the wave function (Diosi, 1989; Penrose, 1996). The kinematic argument, phase-averaging, and decoherence are all consistent with the unitary evolution of quantum physics. They are experimentally accessible and proven to be relevant in well-controlled experiments. But none of them includes a qualitative transition between quantum and classical phenomena – only a gradual reduction of the observability of quantum effects. In contrast to that, collapse models, as taught in many modern physics textbooks, postulate a factual and abrupt change between quantum and classical dynamics, but also this assumption leaves many experimental and philosophical questions unanswered. Also from this fundamental point of view, it is therefore still open to question to which degree quantum physics can prevail on the macroscopic scale of living species.

Can quantumness survive in biological environments? The observation of quantum phenomena often requires low temperatures and a high degree of isolation. And yet, quantum coherence could be observed in matter-wave experiments with bio-dyes even at internal temperatures exceeding 690 K. Related experiments, however, also quantified the high sensitivity of quantum coherence to the emission or scattering of even single photons or molecules (Hornberger et al., 2003). A simple and general rule reads as follows: if an individual state of a quantum superposition can be resolved and detected by any interaction with its environment, the superposition will be destroyed. A practical example: a molecule that coherently traverses several slits of a diffraction grating will maintain its quantum superposition until the environment gets the capability of reading which slit the particle takes.

Even if the openings are separated by only 250 nm, the scattering of a single visible photon per molecule may destroy the observation of quantum interference. Under biological conditions, in an aqueous and warm environment, position superpositions of massive particles cannot survive more than a few collisions with electrons, atoms, photons, or phonons. In the case of strong interactions, a single collision will destroy the coherence. And even for weak perturbations, the visibility of quantum phenomena will vanish exponentially with the separation of the position states. Any delocalization in biomaterials will therefore be limited to extensions of a few nanometers and time scales typically shorter than nanoseconds, in most cases only a few hundred femtoseconds. But a few backdoors still exists for coherence and entanglement to persist: first, it is conceivable that special molecular architectures may shield some parts of a system from some interactions with their environment. Electrostatic forces may, for instance, create hydrophobic pockets from which the solvent could be excluded. But the existence and survival of decoherence-free subspaces (Lidar et al., 1998) in organic matter and over the time scales of milliseconds still has to be shown experimentally. Secondly, quantum error correction (Shor, 1995) is often being discussed as a loophole for the implementation of quantum information processing in living systems. The idea is based on the fact that a certain class of computational errors may even be corrected if no one knows the details of the state or the errors that occurred. This is particularly important, as any attempt to read a quantum superposition would result in its loss, i.e. its reduction to a classical state. A system with quantum error correction requires, however, even more qubits than the uncoded counterpart. The idea of the scheme has been demonstrated with a 3-bit code in NMR quantum computing with alanine (Cory et al., 1998), but as of today, extensions to more than a handful of spins at low temperatures are not known. We thus face the following dilemma: what are the odds that quantum error correction was developed by natural selection from unprotected quantum computing if a faulty precursor process would provide no evolutionary advantage?

Finally, it is worth noting that biology operates in open systems, i.e. far from thermal equilibrium. It has been hypothesized that living systems might act as heat engines, providing local cooling in an otherwise thermal environment (Matsuno, 1999). Another perspective (Cai et al., 2008) puts forth the hypothesis that entanglement might be regularly refreshed in a thermally driven, repetitive contact between neighboring molecular subsystems. If that happens on a timescale shorter than the one of decoherence, net entanglement may possibly persist. Clearly, all of these ideas are presently of an exploratory nature.

How can quantum entanglement be revealed in mesoscopic systems? We introduced entanglement as the inseparability of quantum states. But how could we possibly detect this intricate quantumness in a complex condensed matter environment, where there is no hope of getting access to all underlying details? Interestingly, it has been found, that even macroscopic thermodynamical variables may serve as entanglement witnesses (Vedral, 2003; Amico et al., 2008). And to a certain degree, entanglement may even survive in a macroscopic thermal state (Markham et al., 2008). Since the Hamiltonian, i.e. the operator of the system's total energy, that is used for deriving all thermodynamic functions is influenced by the entanglement of the underlying wave functions, the energy terms and therefore also all thermodynamic variables are affected by these quantum correlations. A single macroscopic observable phenomenon can thus suffice to hint to the presence of quantum entanglement, while the important trick is to find an observable that can be reliably read in experiments. In practice, the magnetic susceptibility (Brukner et al., 2006) or the heat capacity might provide good indicators for entanglement and it will be interesting to search for further witnesses in biological systems as well. There is an enormous reduction of information when we derive a single thermodynamical variable from thousands of quantum states. Entanglement witnesses therefore cannot tell us all details about a system. They rather indicate under which conditions a state is definitely entangled, but they neither quantify it nor do they exclude with certainty the presence of entanglement if the witness conditions are violated.

Life Science Research with an Interface to Quantum Physics

Single-photon phenomena in the life sciences. Single quanta of light have been relevant for illustrating fundamental quantum principles but they are also ubiquitous in the life sciences. The most efficient detection techniques for fluorescent biomolecules are sensitive on the single photon level. Individual particles of light are also of direct relevance in biological processes as they may affect the structure of individual molecules which in turn can transduce signals in living organisms. The retinal molecule can switch its conformation after absorption of very few photons and thus turns the human eye into one of the most sensitive light-detecting devices that exists. Between two and seven photons are usually sufficient to be perceived by a dark-adapted human observer (Hecht et al., 1942). Various studies indicated that test persons could even count the number of photons with a reliability that was only limited by quantum shot noise (Rieke and Baylor, 1998, and citations therein). Single photon detectors are of great interest for quantum communication and it has recently been suggested that octopus rhodopsin, chosen by evolution because it is well-adapted to the dark of the deep oceans, may be a useful component in such applications (Sivozhelezov and Nicolini, 2007). But furthermore, single photon sources are gaining increasing importance in quantum communication or computation protocols and single molecules are considered to be relevant emitters (Lounis and Orrit, 2005).

When we talk about the quantum properties of light, we usually refer to its wave-particle duality, the graininess and quantum statistical properties, such as photon bunching, anti-bunching, or squeezing (Glauber, 2006). Fluorescence correlation experiments with proteins (Sanchez-Mosteiro et al., 2004) have revealed both the discrete quantum nature of molecular energy states and the non-thermal quantum statistics of light. An excited single molecule may usually not absorb a second photon of identical wavelength unless the excited state has decayed. The emitted photons are therefore released with a time structure which differs from that of thermal light sources. Photons emitted by a single molecule come in an anti-bunched rather than a bunched time series. It remains, however, still open whether single-photon emission is explicitly used by living systems. In contrast to that, artificially-grown quantum emitters have found many applications in the life sciences. The characteristic energy of a quantum system is connected with its spatial dimensions. This is particularly true for semiconductor nanocrystals, which measure only a few nanometers in diameter and whose color can be changed from blue to red by growing them to larger sizes. Fluorescent quantum dots are used as highly-efficient labels for biomolecular imaging and they allow researchers to follow the dynamics of marked receptors in the neural membrane of living cells (Dahan et al., 2003). Similar results have recently also been achieved with nanodiamonds. Their nitrogen vacancy centers exhibit strong and stable fluorescence, they are biocompatible, and they have also been proven to be highly-sensitive quantum probes for magnetic fields on the nanoscale (e.g. Balasubramanian et al., 2008).

Quantum tunneling in biomolecules: from enzymatic reactions to the olfactory sense? Living organisms are enormous biochemical reactors, making and breaking zillions of chemical bonds every day. To a large extent, the reaction rates are controlled both by thermal activation and enzymatic catalysis. It has been a long-standing question whether quantum tunneling is also involved and whether its presence provides an evolutionary advantage. This concerns the tunneling of electrons, protons, and even entire small molecules. The theory of electron transfer has a long history (Marcus, 1956). First, evidence for electron tunneling was derived from the oxidation rate of cytochrome (see Figure 3b) in the bacterium chromatium vinosum. Since the reaction speeds were both large and temperature independent at low temperatures (<100 K), it was concluded that they are incompatible with a thermal activation model alone (De Vault and Chance, 1966). Electron tunneling has actually been identified as a widespread process, found in photosynthesis (Blankenship, 1989), cellular respiration (Gray and Winkler, 2003), and electron transport along DNA (Winkler et al., 2005). While speculations about proton tunneling had also been around for long (Löwdin, 1963), first experimental evidence was only given in 1989 (Cha et al., 1989) for the enzyme alcohol dehydrogenase, which transfers a proton from alcohol to nicotinamide adenine dinucleotide. Since tunneling depends on the mass of the object, the tunneling rates must change when hydrogen is replaced by the chemically-equivalent deuterium which doubles the atomic mass. This kinetic isotope effect was confirmed and gives good evidence for the presence of proton tunneling. Since then, many other enzymatic reactions were ascribed to proton tunneling (Glickman et al., 1994). It has to be noted, however, that the tunneling distances involved in all these reactions are typically shorter than 0.1 nm and the protons traverse the barrier at energies around 10 kcal/mol (0.4 eV) below the potential maximum (Masgrau et al., 2006). The simultaneous tunneling of several particles has also been discussed, including double, triple, and even quadruple proton exchange in cyclic molecular networks (Brougham et al., 1999). The transition rates in these experiments were measured using NMR spectroscopy and the temperature dependence of the reaction rate as well as the kinetic isotope effect were taken as witnesses for the presence of hydrogen tunneling. Even the tunneling of entire small molecules, i.e. formaldehyde (CH2 O), was proposed based on the temperature dependence of its photo-induced polymerization rate (Goldanskii, 1979). Turin (1996) also opened a public debate by suggesting that we are even able to smell quantum tunneling. Most aspects of our sense of smell are very well-understood without it. Linda Buck and Richard Axel received the Nobel Prize for their description of the mammalian olfactory system. They identified transmembrane proteins that encode for odor receptors in the olfactory epithelium (Buck and Axel, 1991). Each of them can sense multiple odorants. And each odorant can be detected by different sensors. Most smells can be perfectly explained (Zarzo, 2007) by assuming a lock-and-key mechanism, where an odor molecule binds to a specific receptor combination depending on its size, shape, and chemical groups.

Based on much earlier hypotheses (Dyson, 1938), Turin suggested that smell is, at least additionally, correlated to the vibrational spectrum of molecules and that the receptors perform phonon-assisted inelastic electron tunneling spectroscopy to identify the odorant. This idea should explain why our nose is able to distinguish molecular groups of similar geometry but different vibrational spectra, such as, for example, OH and SH or ferrocene and nickelocene (Turin, 2002). However, recent experiments (Keller and Vosshall, 2004) rejected this theory, while newer theoretical work conceded a conceptual viability of the idea – even though it was not quantitatively decisive (Brookes et al., 2007). Concluding, we see that quantum tunneling is certainly present in a large number of biological processes, but experimentally proven only on the level of small-scale chemical reactions.

Coherent excitation transfer in photosynthesis. Photosynthesis is a key process for life and often considered as a role model for future light harvesting technologies (Blankenship, 2002). It is differently realized in plants, algae, and bacteria, but they all convert light to chemical energy. A closer consideration reveals that photosynthesis involves a plethora of highly-complex processes, such as long-ranged excitation transfer, redox-reactions, hydrolysis, proton transport, or phosphorylation. In many parts of the system – including the wet-chemical material transport – we don't expect to find significant quantum coherence or entanglement, but others may actually require the notion of quantum tunneling, coherent excitonic transfer, or matter-wave interference. The photosynthetic complex is a membrane-bound system with many embedded functional subunits. The energy conversion starts with the absorption of an incident photon by a pigment molecule, e.g. a chlorophyll, porphyrin, or a carotenoid molecule embedded in a protein structure, the antenna complex. The large number of these dye units ensures a high photoabsorption probability, and their arrangement enables an efficient excitation transfer from the primary absorber to the reaction center. The reaction center is a pigment-protein complex which contains a dimer, called the special pair. When it is excited, it donates an electron to a neighboring acceptor molecule. Fast secondary processes prevent the recombination of the ion pair and trigger the release of protons that are first transferred across the membrane and later used to fuel – for instance, the synthesis of adenosine triphosphate (ATP) from adenosine diphosphate (ADP). Several recent studies (van Grondelle and Novoderezhkin, 2006; Cheng and Fleming, 2009) emphasized how well the excitation transfer from the antenna pigments to the reaction center is optimized. A fast conversion is important, since any delay would increase the chances of relaxation mechanisms to channel energy into heating instead of chemical potentials. Early explanations of the energy transport, based on incoherent and dipole-dipole-mediated excitation hopping between molecular sites (Förster, 1948), failed to explain the observed transfer rates. Delocalization and coherent exciton coupling between the closely-packed antenna pigments were therefore suggested as the most likely explanation, with experimental support rapidly growing throughout recent years. Modern two-dimensional Fourier transform spectroscopy allowed researchers to probe the various excitation transfer pathways between the molecules on a femtosecond time scale. In particular, experiments performed on a 77 K temperature bacteriochlorophyll Fenna–Matthews–Olsen antenna complex were able to reveal exciton delocalization (Brixner et al., 2005) and long-lasting coherence in the excitonic energy transfer observation of a spatially- and temporally-extended coherence, covering several nanometers and timespans as long as a few hundred femtoseconds, is highly remarkable and it has triggered a growing number of scientific groups to focus their theoretical and experimental work on that question. As of today, a rich set of detailed data has already been collected to characterize the energy levels, transfer rates, intramolecular and intermolecular coherences. In particular, the latter raised the question of how to connect these findings to related fields in quantum physics. When there is coherence, what is the role of constructive or destructive interference? And are we allowed to use the language of quantum information processing to describe the highly-efficient natural transfer of information and energy in light-harvesting complexes? It has been suggested that a wavelike sampling of the energy landscape or even a quantum search algorithm might permit us to find the fastest route from the antenna to the reaction center (Engel et al., 2007). The excitation transport has also been associated with quantum random walks (Mohseni et al., 2008). In contrast to classical random walks – which we also know from Brownian motion – the position of the quantum walker would not be a single random position, but rather a superposition of positions. The incorporation of interference effects in the theoretical reasoning led to further considerations concerning the possible role of the protein environment (Rebentrost et al., 2009; Olaya-Castro et al., 2008), since a close look at wave physics reveals that coherence can be both beneficial and a hindrance if the aim is to optimize the speed of transport. On the one hand, the simultaneous wavelike sampling of many parallel paths could possibly result in finding a faster way to the final goal. But on the other hand, the presence of an irregular lattice of scattering centers (static disorder) may actually suppress wave transport because of destructive interference. This phenomenon, well know in solid state physics, is called Anderson localization (Anderson, 1958). In that case, thermal fluctuations of the protein environment might, therefore, be crucial and help to avoid localization, and thus assist in the excitation transfer (Caruso et al., 2009). The importance of protein dynamics in eliminating Anderson localization was actually already discussed in an earlier paper by (Balabin and Onuchic, 2000), where multiple quantum pathways and interferences were proposed for the electron transfer. The role of interference in transport phenomena can also be visualized by recalling the analogy to an optical Mach-Zehnder interferometer (as shown in Figure 1d). Depending on the setting of phases, wave interference can guide all excitations to either one of the two exits. Quantum coherence may then be the best way to channel the interfering quanta to the desired output. But if the wave phases happened to be initially-set to destructive interference, quantum coherence would be a severe handicap. In this case, even random dephasing processes would help to optimize the transport efficiency.

External perturbations may also be important for energetic reasons: the electronic excitations have to be transferred between complexes of different energy. If the molecular states were too well-defined, the lacking energy overlap would reduce the transfer rate. External perturbations may broaden the transition bands and thus increase the coupling between neighboring molecules. Recent experiments by Collini and Scholes (2009), however, hint also at another possible role of the protein environment. In their experiments they showed that coherent electronic excitation transfer along conjugated polymer chains occurs even at room temperature. These long-lasting coherences (200 fs) could only be observed in intrachain, but not in interchain, electronic excitation transfers. All of the models described above bear in common that they rely on quantum coherence and decoherence and that they may be robust even under ambient environmental conditions over short time scales. It is thus the fine interplay of coherent exciton transfer, decoherence, and dephasing that yields the best results and which seems to reign one of the most important reactions in nature.

Conformational quantum superpositions in biomolecules. Since atoms can exist in a superposition of position states, this may also lead to a superposition of conformational states in molecules. A tunneling-induced superposition of conformation states is conceivable. It becomes, however, highly-improbable when many atoms have to be shifted over large distances and across high potential wells during the state change. Photo-isomerization is another way of inducing structural state changes in molecules now using photon exchange instead of tunneling. This opens the possibility to connect even energetically-separated states. The photo-induced all-trans–13-cis transition of retina is a famous example where a single photon can cause a sizeable conformation change. But much of the subsequent atom rearrangement occurs in interactions with the thermal environment (Gai et al., 1998). In spite of that, it was possible to gain coherent quantum control in this process. Applying pulse-shaped femtosecond laser excitation to retinal in a native protein environment (Prokhorenko et al., 2006) achieved a modulation of the isomerization yield by ±20 %. The detected dependence on the laser phase is a good indication for the relevance of quantum interference among vibrational states. But a coherent superposition of functionally-different configuration states, instead of electronic or vibrational states, has not yet been achieved for any large biomolecule.

Decoherence has often been named to explain the prevalence of chirality in biomolecules. If a molecule may exist in two enantiomers, quantum mechanics allows, in principle, also for a coherent superposition of the left-handed and the right-handed states. In practice, however, this is not observed for larger particles. An intuitive argument is based on the fact that various scattering processes between a molecule and its environment depend on its chirality. This may include the scattering of polar light and elementary particles or the interaction through higher-order London dispersive forces between polarizable bodies. Such events may act as quantum measurements and projections onto a chirality state. And in many cases, the energy barrier between the symmetric ground states will then be too high to allow for their spontaneous mixing on a time scale comparable to the scattering events (Trost and Hornberger, 2009). The generation and controlled decoherence of chirality superposition states in biological molecules thus still remains an open challenge. The lack of any experimental evidence for coherent conformation superpositions in large molecules also seriously questions a recent model by Hameroff and Penrose who suggested that the collapse of such superpositions in microtubuli may be the cause for the emergence of human consciousness (Hameroff and Penrose, 1996).

Spin and the magnetic orientation of migratory birds. It is well established that various animals are able to derive direction information from the geomagnetic field (Wiltschko and Wiltschko, 1995; Ritz et al., 2000; Johnsen and Lohmann, 2008). Some mammals perceive the Earth's field as a polarity compass, distinguishing North and South, while birds and reptiles rely on an inclination compass that discriminates between pole-wards and equator-wards and which exploits both the intensity and the gradient of the field. Interestingly, it can be shown (Wiltschko and Wiltschko, 2006 and refs. therein) that the orientation in the magnetic field requires the presence of visible light beyond a certain photon energy and that an oscillating magnetic field (0.1-10 MHz) can disturb the bird's senses. It has therefore been argued that vision-based magnetosensing might be rooted in the light-induced formation of a radical pair (Schulten et al., 1978), a mechanism originally invoked to explain the photochemically-induced dynamic polarization in nuclei (Closs, 1969; Kaptein and Oosterhoff, 1969). When light falls onto a donor molecule in the bird's eye, it may excite it to a singlet state (Figure 3c). The molecule may then transfer an electron to a neighboring acceptor molecule. The freshly-formed pair of radical molecules usually starts in a singlet state (total spin quantum number: s=0), but in the presence of hyperfine couplings with the molecular nuclei, it will undergo an inter-conversion between the singlet and the triplet state (s=1). Since spin is otherwise rather well-protected from environmental influences on a short timescale, it is assumed that the spin pair remains quantum correlated, i.e. entangled in this process. This is also supported by a recent calculation (Rieper et al., 2009), where even a weak external oscillatory magnetic field noise was admitted and not able to fully destroy entanglement. The evolution of the electron spins both in the presence of the nuclei and the earth's magnetic field will vary the ratio between singlet and triplet states. Since many chemical reactions are spin-dependent – in particular, also the back-transfer of the electron from the acceptor to the donor – the spin evolution should also influence the ratio of molecular products that are finally formed in the bird's eye. A model for the transduction from the radical pair to the neuronal correlates was proposed by Weaver et al. (2000), who also estimated the requirements on the size and the temperature dependence of the system in order to yield a certain sensitivity. The radical pair mechanism was ascribed to the signalling protein cryptochrome that can be found in the bird's retina (Wiltschko and Wiltschko, 2006). Both the electron transfer from a photo-excited flavin adenine dinucleotide along a chain of tryptophan molecules and the reverse recombination reaction are supposed to be sensitive to the geomagnetic field (Solov'yov and Schulten, 2009).

The idea is further supported by recent experiments of Maeda et al. (2008), who showed that the radical pair mechanism in the earth's field is actually sufficiently strong to alter the chemical end products in a custom-designed complex that was built from a carotenoid, a porphyrin, and a fullerene C60. In order to further corroborate that magneto-sensing is related to quantum-correlated (entangled) electrons, Cai et al. (2009) suggested the use of a sequence of short radio-frequency pulses to obtain active quantum control over the radical pair spins, immediately after their creation. Such and related experiments are still required to further elucidate this intriguing phenomenon.

Speculations on quantum information and biology on the large scale. Most puzzles of quantum physics are related to the way information is encoded and processed. Some researchers would therefore demand that quantum biology should be defined by its use of quantum information. The present section recapitulates two recent speculations which aim at much larger scales than that of a few molecules. We clearly state that, as of today, these hypotheses are without any experimental justification and are even disputed on theoretical grounds. But, as some of them have gained rather high popularity in discussions, they merit mentioning and brief comments.

Quantum physics and the human mind. About two decades ago, Roger Penrose raised the question of whether classical physics alone could suffice to explain the enormous problem-solving capabilities of the human brain (Penrose, 1989). He speculated that a combination of currently irreconcilable pieces of physics, namely quantum theory and general relativity, might open a new window to our understanding of human consciousness, i.e. another phenomenon which is hardly understood. Together with the consciousness scientist Stuart Hameroff, he proposed a model that assumes that the human mind may exploit at least two conformations of microtubuli as values of a quantum bit. The quan- tumness of the proteins was suggested to solve complex computational problems in the brain while the act of consciousness would be linked to a gravity-induced objective collapse of the quantum wave function (Hameroff and Penrose, 1996). Intriguing as the idea of macroscopic quantum coherence may be, the proposed model hits several hard bounds and controversies. As of today, no one has ever been able to prepare and characterize a useful coherent macroscopic quantum superposition of two conformations in a macromolecule, not even in a laboratory. And even if it existed in nature, decoherence is believed to be orders of magnitude too fast to make it relevant on physiological timescales (Tegmark, 2000; Eisert and Wiseman, 2007). An objective collapse of the wave function is currently also only one of many models to explain the emergence of classicality from quantum physics. The dynamics of the proposed gravitational collapse is neither theoretically-understood nor experimentally-observed. It may also be surprising that microtubuli were chosen as the decisive agents in quantum consciousness. They are by no means specific to the human brain, but are rather ubiquitous cell support structures. In spite of its potential deficiencies, the model serves a purpose in that it stretches the scientific fantasy to its very limits. And even though it is unlikely that all details of the proposal will survive future scientific explorations, experimental efforts, in proving or disproving these details, will lead to new insights regarding the relevance of quantum phenomena within the life sciences.

Quantum aspects of the brain waves. If highly-transient neuron assemblies are indeed a key feature of the brain operations that cause consciousness, a critical issue—for scientists, especially—is how they might actually be formed. The idea developed in this book is that, because we have only one consciousness at any one moment (Arieli, 1995), the dominant assembly for that moment would have to be so massive that it precluded the formation of any other sufficiently large rivals—the recruitment of, say, 10^7 neurons in less than 250 milli-seconds. However, even this large number is simply the response of a group of neurons to a flash of light and does not necessarily entail consciousness. The requisite size of an appropriate neuron assembly might be far greater still.

Classical synaptic transmission is perfectly adequate for coordinating the firing of a million or so neurons in a fraction of a second. It is important to remember that neuron firing of an action potential is not linear, with one domino causing the fall of its neighbor, one at a time. Yet, if the firing of one neuron causes *N* neighbors to fire, then after *S* steps, $-N^5$ neurons will fire in a huge three-dimensional domino effect. Even if *N* were as small as 10, only 6 steps would be needed to assemble a million neurons.

But suppose that synaptic transmission is not, after all, doing the job. According to the calculations, the spread of activity from the epicenter activated by the flash of light is some 100 to 250 cm/s. This is much faster than a wave of seizure in epilepsy (1 cm/s), yet it is actually much slower than classic synaptic signaling, where an action potential can be propagated down the neuron axon at speeds of up to 10,000 cm/s. Whereas classic synaptic signaling is useful in local circuits of neurons, perhaps a different process is operational in the more gradual recruitment of very large, global assemblies that will in turn be necessary for consciousness.

A synapse is a highly-specialized point of contact, as different from a mere gap as riverboat stations are from featureless banks facing each other across the water (Levitan and Kaczmarek, 1996). A simpler but less-specialized system involves the mere fusion of one dendrite of one cell with that of another, so that electrical current spreads passively, without the need for a participating chemical. These points of fusion are called "gap junctions." Perhaps the spread of activation through the agency of gap junctions is what distinguishes the formation of a very large neuronal assembly. In support of this idea, John Jefferys and his colleagues have confirmed that the much-studied oscillations of some 40 Hz are generated as a result of normal synaptic transmission. What is particularly intriguing, however, is that Jefferys has also shown that it is possible for neurons to work collectively at a much faster rate, that there are, in addition, much faster oscillations of some 200 Hz. This higher-frequency orchestration is mediated not by synapses but by gap junctions. (Draguhn, 1998).

Perhaps the very extensive type of neuron assembly that mediates consciousness will be composed of synchronous neuron firing at a frequency far higher than the much-studied 40 Hz. However, because this type of activity depends on coherent gap junction signaling—which is less efficient than classic synaptic transmission—the time taken for large numbers of neurons to be recruited into a synchronous, large-scale assembly will be slower—the good half a second observed. These features—relatively slow-to-form, yet high-frequency coherence once established—might be advantageous in first stabilizing a moment of consciousness, and second in optimizing conditions for a very high-frequency firing so that the signature peptide profile can then be released.

Another alternative to the traditional picture involves a very different mechanism that might operate at a much more minuscule level, beyond the cell itself, and beyond the classic physics of Newton which is successful for describing events in the everyday world, and with it, in principle at least, traditional neuroscience. Just such a vision has captured the imagination of the mathematician Roger Penrose and the anesthetist Stuart Hameroff (Hameroff, Penrose, 2003). Their version of events does not rely on the classic generation of action potentials, but rather on a faster and far more speculative process that is based on quantum theory.

Penrose and Hameroff's speculations about the nature of consciousness begin by noting that in one interpretation of quantum theory, the very act of observation causes a system to be in one type of unpredictable state, a phenomenon they call "subjective reduction." It is subjective because it requires an observer. In the brain, however, there is no outside observer, and hence the appropriate conditions might prevail under which quantum events are not downgraded subjectively, but rather occur spontaneously, without anyone watching. This hypothetical phenomenon has been called objective reduction (OR) by Penrose and Hameroff, who believe that the concept of OR could underpin a new type of physics. Because OR would not obey the computable and established rules of either quantum physics or Newtonian physics, they consider that this new physics would be most appropriate for generating consciousness—another incomputable phenomenon.

Quantum theory offers the appropriate time and space scales for assembling millions of neurons in a fraction of a second into a working assembly. This procedure is known as quantum coherence. However, we have seen that classical processes can proceed just as well. Yet here too, in quantum coherence, there might be a good candidate for a neural correlate of consciousness.

Penrose and Hameroff have speculated that the medium of such orchestration could be the tiny, fluid-filled microtubules, which are present in virtually every cell in the body. Coherence would occur, they suggest, by exciting water molecules buried in a protein called *tubulin*, the building block of microtubules. Tubulin can undergo conformational changes in molecular structure. The idea stipulates that these changes could support wavelike signals propagated in accord with quantum theory, from which comes Penrose and Hameroff's speculation: once the number of neurons is sufficiently large, then, in accord with the as yet nonexistent *New Physics*, there would be a spontaneous downgrading of the wave, an OR across large numbers of cells. This OR, a sudden commitment to one type of physical state, would somehow correspond to a moment of consciousness in the macro brain.

As it stands, the existence of microtubules and the idea of quantum coherence as a basis for consciousness has not so much been shown to be wrong, but on its own, it has simply been unhelpful for biologists—it is too abstract to be usefully applied to the tangible brain, and it is without experimental motivation.

For Penrose and Hameroff's idea to qualify as a successful correlate of consciousness, three basic issues still need to be resolved before biologists can make use of it. First, we need a further feature to the scheme whereby the number of requisite coherent neurons can be increased from the tens and hundreds of thousands, to tens and hundreds of millions. Second, a means of accounting for the role of chemically-diverse transmitter systems is needed. Third, we need a reason for discriminating between certain microtubules, such that only those in certain neurons, and not in just any old cell, are appropriate to mediate consciousness at certain times.

One possible way of overcoming these problems lies in a scheme advanced by the neuroscientist Woolf (1975). Woolf's model starts off conventionally-enough. Neurons in a certain brain region, the *basal forebrain,* are active and release the transmitter acetylcholine, in the accepted fashion, on to neurons in the cortex. Acetylcholine will, again in the traditional way, act via its normal molecular targets, its receptors, on discrete modules of neurons, stretching some 1 to 2 mm^2 in the cortex. But now some of the consequences might be unexpected: in addition to its action within local circuitry, Woolf has suggested a chemical-selective and site-selective means whereby the quantum coherence based on microtubule operations could be set in train.

Models such as the one we have just explored, based on Woolf's imaginative exploitation of the known actions of MAP2 and acetylcholine, are, at the very least, useful in that they cross the traditional disciplines of physics and neuroscience to show how a combination of phenomena, rules, and constraints from each can make a more robust and plausible model.

Note that this hybrid theory is once again dependent on good old-fashioned transmitter signaling. We cannot rule out the possibility that acetylcholine—as a prototype neurochemical—plays an important role in triggering other, non-classical events as well as at the more macro level of brain function – for example, as a neuromodulator, putting cells on red alert. All the electrical signals are generated in the same rhythm of oscillations. However, no single cell joins in all the activity all the time, but overall, there are sufficient cells to maintain a synchronous activity for very long periods of time. Acetylcholine in this instance has enabled a whole population of cells to become more important than the individual units.

Whatever the eventual mechanisms of attaining a transient coherence in a very large assembly of neurons turn out to be, there is no shortage of candidates, even at the moment. The future will no doubt reveal more, along with means for testing which ones really do play a part in the formation of assemblies, and hence in the reality of a neural correlate of consciousness that is not just necessary but sufficient.

Classical theory of brain waves. How does the brain differ from the heart, liver, and other organs? All organ systems are enormously complicated structures, able to repair themselves, and make detailed responses to external control by chemical or electrical input. Yet, only brains yield the amazing phenomenon of consciousness (Nunez, 2010). Complex adaptive systems, for which human brains provide the most prominent examples, are composed of smaller parts interacting both within and across spatial scales. They typically exhibit emergent behavior that is not obviously predictable from knowledge of the individual parts and have the added capacity to learn from experience and change their global behaviors by means of feedback processes. Other examples include stock markets, ecosystems, and all living systems.

Several general features distinguish human brains from other organs, including the hallmark of richer hierarchical (or multi-scale) interactions. In contrast to simple cognitive theories, Nunez's papers explicitly acknowledge brains as highly-complex adaptive systems, emphasizing the critical contribution of cross scale interactions to their dynamic behaviors. In order to minimize communication barriers due to the complicated mathematics, several analog systems from disparate fields are employed. Neuroscientists are typically skeptical of brain analogs, typically for good reason; however, we are *not* claiming that brains are actually just like stretched strings, social systems, quantum structures, resonant cavities, hot plasmas, disordered solids, chaotic fluids, or any other non-neural system.

In many complex systems, as spatial-temporal scales of observation are increased, new phenomena become evident by virtue of synergistic interactions among smaller-scale entities, which serve to explain data, typically in a mathematically-aesthetic fashion. For example, in the classical thermodynamics of equilibrium systems, it is possible to transition from microscopic molecular scales to macroscopic scales and employ the macroscopic variable temperature to describe the average kinetic energy of microscopic molecular activity. Many complex systems, however, operate in non-equilibrium states, being driven by nonlinear and stochastic interactions. For such systems, classical thermodynamics typically do not apply. For example, the description of weather and ocean patterns, which includes important features such as turbulence, rely on semi-phenomenological mesoscopic models, in agreement with molecular theories but not capable of being rigorously derived from them. Phase transitions in magnetic systems and many systems similarly modeled require careful treatment of a continuum of scales near critical points. In general, rather than having a general theory of non-equilibrium nonlinear process, several overlapping approaches are employed, typically geared to classes of systems and often expanding on nonlinear treatments of stochastic systems (Gardiner, 1983). Given this general outline of complex systems, it should not be surprising that human brains support many phenomena arising at different spatial-temporal scales. One can study macroscopic neocortical phenomena such as electroencephalography

(EEG) by appealing to a chain of arguments dealing with overlapping microscopic and mesoscopic scales. Such work is detailed in a series of papers presenting a theory of statistical mechanics of neocortical interactions (Ingber & Nunez, 1990). This approach permits us to develop EEG and other models of dynamic processes whose variables and parameters are closely identified with ensembles of synaptic and neuronal interactions. The mathematical formalism supporting this approach has only recently been made possible by developments in mathematical physics since the late 1970s, in the field of nonlinear non-equilibrium statistical mechanics. The origins of this theory are in quantum and gravitational field theory.

EEG allows for accurate identification of distinct sleep stages, depth of anesthesia, seizures, and other neurological disorders. It also reveals robust correlations with cognitive processes occurring during mental calculations, working memory, and selective attention. Scientists are now so accustomed to these EEG correlations with brain states such that they may forget just how remarkable they are. The scalp EEG provides very large-scale and robust measures of neocortical dynamic function. A single electrode yields estimates of synaptic action averaged over tissue masses containing between roughly 100 million and 1 billion neurons. The space averaging of brain potentials resulting from extra-cranial recording is a fortuitous data reduction process forced by current spreading in the head volume conductor. Much more detailed local information may be obtained from intracranial recordings in animals and epileptic patients. However, intracranial electrodes implanted in living brains provide only very sparse spatial coverage, thereby failing to record the “big picture” of brain function. Furthermore, the dynamic behavior of intracranial recordings depends fundamentally on measurement scale, determined mostly by electrode size. Different electrode sizes and locations can result in substantial differences in recorded dynamic behavior, including frequency content and coherence. Thus, in practice, intracranial data provide different information, not more information, than is obtained from the scalp (Nunez, Srinivasan, 2006a).

In practice, intracranial EEG may be uncorrelated or only weakly-correlated with cognition and behavior. The information content in such recordings is limited by sparse spatial sampling and scale-dependent dynamics. Furthermore, most intracranial EEG data are recorded in lower mammals; extrapolation to humans involves additional issues. Thus, higher brain function in humans is more easily observed at large scales. Scientists interested in higher brain function are fortunate in this respect. The technical and ethical limitations of human intracranial recording force us to emphasize scalp recordings. These extra-cranial recordings provide estimates of synaptic action at the large scales closely related to cognition and behavior. Thus, EEG provides a window on the mind, albeit one that is often clouded by technical and other limitations.

Since the first human recording in the early 1920s, the physiological bases for the wide variety of rhythmic EEG activity, a proverbial “spectral zoo,” has been somewhat of a mystery. In particular, human alpha rhythms, which are quite robust in wide awake (but relaxed) subjects with closed eyes, may be recorded over nearly all of the upper scalp or cortex and have preferred frequencies near 10 Hz. Given any unknown physical or biological system that produces oscillations at some preferred (or resonant) frequency $f = \omega / 2\pi$, one of the first questions a scientist might ask concerns the origin of the implied underlying time delay $\boldsymbol{x}$ roughly estimated as

$$\tau = \omega^{-1} \quad (1)$$

The implied physiological time scales for the most robust human EEG rhythms (1 to 15 Hz) are t = 10 -160 ms. How does this delay range compare with mammalian physiology? Whereas early studies of membrane time constants in the mammalian cortex were very short, typically less than 10 ms, more modern studies with improved recording methods report the wide range 20 -100 ms. But apparently in voltage-gated channels, the effective time constant becomes a "dynamical parameter" that depends on both membrane voltage and on time, thus genuine time constants are not really "constant." Koch (2004) argues that the voltage response to very brief synaptic inputs is essentially independent of the classically-defined time constant, which typically provides overestimates of the response time of neurons. In summary, these studies suggest that while synaptic delays (PSP rise and decay times) lie in a general range (within a factor of perhaps five or ten) that might account for dominant EEG frequencies, claims of close agreement between the details of observed EEG spectra and dynamic theories based on membrane time constants are not credible. Model parameters can be chosen to "match" favored EEG data sets, which, in any case, can vary widely between individuals and brain states.

In contrast to these "local" delays at the single neuron level, axonal ("global") delays along the (corticocortical) fibers between anterior and posterior regions are estimated to be roughly in the 30 ms range in humans (Nunez, 1995). Such global delays depend on axon length distribution and axon propagation speed; thus, they are expected to be much shorter in smaller mammalian brains if axon diameters (or propagation speed) are unchanged across species. To complicate matters, creation of serial connections between cell assemblies can apparently modify both local (PSP) and global (axon) characteristic delay times. While both local and global delays appear to be in a general range favorable for EEG production, this semi-quantitative observation tells us little about the physiological mechanisms responsible for "special frequencies" like the narrow band human alpha rhythms or gamma oscillations (about 40 Hz), the latter recorded mostly from inside the craniums of humans and lower mammals. Neither local theories (based on PSP rise and decay times) nor global theories (based on axon delays) can honestly claim close agreement with EEG data based *only* on predicted EEG spectral properties; the underlying physiological parameters (e.g., time constants and axonal delays) are not known with sufficient accuracy to make such claims credible. While PN Nunez has suggested that the parameters of the global standing wave theory appear to be known more accurately than local parameters, others may disagree. Nevertheless, we *can* agree to search for qualitative and semi-quantitative connections between theory and EEG experiments that do not require precise physiological parameter knowledge.

The general idea of standing EEG waves (Nunez, 1974) was based on a very simple idea. Any kind of weakly-damped, non-dispersive wave phenomenon propagating in a medium with characteristic speed v can be expected to form standing waves due to wave interference that depends on the system's size and shape (the boundary conditions). Such phenomena occur, for example, in violin and piano strings and many other vibrating systems. Whereas waves in strings and flutes are reflected from boundaries, waves in closed systems, like spherical shells or tori, interfere because of periodic boundary conditions causing waves traveling in opposing directions to meet and combine. As a result of this interference, preferred (resonant) frequencies persist in such systems. Examples of standing waves in spherical geometry include the quantum wave function of the hydrogen atom (both radial and tangential waves) and the Schumann resonances of electromagnetic waves in the spherical shell formed by the earth's surface and the bottom of the ionosphere (tangential waves only). The lowest frequency, often dominant in such systems, is the fundamental mode. This fundamental frequency is given for the geometries of a spherical shell of radius R or a one dimensional loop of length $L = 2nR$, perhaps a closed loop of transmission line (Nunez, 1995), by

$$f = \frac{gv}{L} \tag{2}$$

Here, the geometric constant g is either β (spherical shell) or 1 (one dimensional loop). Each cortical hemisphere is, topographically, essentially a spherical shell. On the other hand, the postulated medium characteristic speed v is the axon propagation speed in the longer systems of corticocortical axons forming in the white matter layer. Since these fibers may be substantially anisotropic with a preferred anterior-posterior orientation, it is unclear whether the shell or loop model is the most appropriate.

The wrinkled surface of each cortical hemisphere can be reshaped or mentally-inflated (as with a balloon) to create an equivalent spherical shell with effective radius R related to its surface area by the relation

$$R = \sqrt{\frac{A}{4\pi}} \tag{3}$$

Thus, cerebral cortex and its white matter system of (mostly) corticocortical fibers is a system somewhat analogous the earth-ionosphere shell. With a brain hemispheric surface area $A\sim$ 800—1500 cm^2 or, alternately, an anterior-posterior closed cortical loop of $L\sim$ 50—70 cm (ellipsoid-like circumference), and a characteristic corticocortical axon propagation speed of $v\sim$ 600—900 cm/sec (data reviewed from four independent studies in [Nunez, 1995]), the predicted fundamental cortical frequency predicted by the naive application of Eq (2) is then

$$v=2 \text{ to } 26 \text{ Hz} \tag{4}$$

This estimate is "naive" because the fundamental mode frequency depends on both the physical shape and material properties of the wave medium (cortex-white matter). These latter properties determine the dispersive nature of the waves; that is, the precise manner in which waves distort when propagating. Such dispersive properties in the cortex are expected to depend on the nature and interactions of the synaptic and action potential fields. Furthermore, cortical frequency must depend on at least one additional parameter determined by the brain state. Thus, estimates in Eqs. (2) and (4) cannot be expected to represent genuine brain waves, even if the cortex were actually a spherical shell or closed loop; the postulated brain waves are much more likely to be dispersive (if for no other reason than most of nature's waves are dispersive). Furthermore, the expected neural networks of cognitive processing (believed to be embedded in global synaptic wave fields) would be expected to cloud experimental observations of standing wave phenomenon. One may guess that such networks involve thalamocortical interactions that can generate preferred frequencies in several bands, including alpha and gamma. Thus, our scalp potentials may be viewed as some mixture of interacting global and local activity, both of which underlie and are correlated with various cognitive events.

These general ideas do not, by any stretch of the imagination, constitute a theory of the brain; rather, they simply suggest a hypothesis and related experiments to test for *traveling* and *standing brain waves.* If estimate Eq. (4) had been obtained before the discovery of the human alpha rhythm in the 1920s, it would have provided a plausible, testable prediction. The appropriate experimental question would have been, "Can brain states be found in which neural network activity is sufficiently suppressed to allow for observation of simple standing waves?" Such imagined experiments would have found the predicted EEG oscillations in the 8-13 Hz band in relaxed subjects (minimal mental load implying minimal network activity) with closed eyes (minimal visual processing).

If anything, the estimate Eq. (4) is almost *too good,* perhaps raising suspicion by critics that parameter estimates have been fudged to make a good story. But, only two parameters, v and L, are involved in the crude frequency estimate. Even if the cortical area estimate were off by a factor of two, the frequency estimate Eq. (4) would only change by V2. The axon speed estimate is based on the four independent studies reviewed by Nunez (1995). When PN Nunez first proposed the idea in 1972, corticocortical propagation speeds were poorly known. Axon speeds in (myelinated) peripheral axons and intracortical (non-myelinated) axons are roughly ten times faster and ten times slower, respectively, than corticocortical axon speeds. That is, human axon speeds vary over at least three orders of magnitude, depending mainly on axon diameter and myelination. Thus, the observed alpha frequency provided a blind prediction of corticocortical axon speed.

The simple standing brain wave model employs *Galilean idealizations* in which many essential properties of genuine brains are deliberately neglected in order to create a simple, useful model. Galileo modeled falling bodies with no air resistance even though he lacked the technology to make the air go away. Similarly, we may lack the technology to fully suppress the brain networks that might eliminate or obscure standing and traveling brain waves, although some anesthesia states may come close to this goal.

The proposed global model is based mostly on the following idea: scalp potentials (EEG) are generated by synaptic current sources at small scales; each cubic millimeter of cortical tissue contains more than 100 million synapses. In contrast to this small scale activity, EEG data are recorded at macroscopic (centimeter) scales, thereby presenting major problems for network models attempting connections to genuine large scale data. The brain wave model follows the macroscopic dependent variables *action potential and synaptic potential densities* – for example, the number of excitatory synaptic events per square millimeter of cortical surface. All dependent variables are expressed as functions of time and cortical location. The basic approach ignores embedded network activity, although networks have been included (approximately) in more advanced models (Nunez, 1989). The predicted resonance frequencies for standing waves in cortex are:

$$f_n = \frac{v}{L}\sqrt{n^2 - (\frac{\beta\lambda L}{2\pi})^2} \tag{5}$$

The symbols and estimated values are:

v: corticocortical propagation speed (600 - 900 cm/sec).

L: effective front-to-back circumference of one cortical hemisphere after inflation to a smooth surface, roughly the shape of a prolate spheroidal shell or rugby ball (50 - 70 cm).

λ : parameter indicating the fall-off in fiber density with cortical distance for the longest corticocortical fiber system (0.1 - 0.3 cm^{-1}).

β : non-dimensional parameter controlled by neuromodulators; β increases correspond to increased background excitability of the cortex (perhaps from thalamocortical interactions, either chemical or electrical). Wave frequency and damping decrease as (*5*) increases four temporal frequencies (Hz) of fundamental mode *(n* = 1) and overtones *(n* > 1) of standing waves. Does the theoretical *dispersion relation* Eq. (5) have any connection to genuine EEG? Surely nothing so simple can do justice to any complex brain! At best, it may enjoy some approximate connections to brains in their more globally-dominated states, possibly coma, anesthesia, deep sleep, some generalized epileptic states, and the more globally-dominant parts of alpha rhythms. A few experimental predictions rely on this equation, but others follow only from the more general idea of standing and traveling brain waves (Nunez, 2010). Note that this model can provide only relationships not comprehensive explanations of complex physiological processes.

In order to distinguish theories of large-scale neocortical dynamics, we have proposed the label *local theory* to indicate mathematical models of cortical or thalamo-cortical interactions for which cortico-cortical axon propagation delays are assumed to be zero. The underlying timescales in these theories typically originate from membrane time constants giving rise to PSP rise and decay times. Thalamocortical networks are also "local" from the viewpoint of a surface electrode, which cannot distinguish purely cortical from thalamocortical networks. Finally, these theories are "local" in the sense of being independent of global boundary conditions dictated by the size and shape of the cortical-white matter system. By contrast, we adopt the label *global theory* to indicate mathematical models in which delays in the cortico-cortical fibers forming most of the white matter in humans provide the important underlying time scale for the large scale EEG dynamics recorded by scalp electrodes. Periodic boundary conditions are generally essential to global theories because the cortical-white matter system is topologically close to a spherical shell.

While this picture of distinct local and global models grossly oversimplifies expected genuine dynamic behaviors with substantial cross-scale interactions, it provides a convenient entry point to brain complexity. To facilitate our discussion, string displacement is governed by the basic string equation (Nunez, 2010)

$$\frac{\partial^2\Phi}{\partial t^2} - v^2\frac{\partial^2\Phi}{\partial x^2} + [\omega_0^2 + f(\Phi)]\Phi = 0 \tag{6}$$

For the simple case of homogeneous linear springs attached to a homogeneous linear string of length *a* and wave speed *v*, the normal modes of oscillation ω_0 are given by

$$\omega_n^2 = \omega_0^2 + (\frac{n\pi v}{a})^2 \tag{7}$$

In this simple limiting case, the natural oscillation frequencies are seen as having distinct local and global contributions given by the first and second terms on the right side of the last equation, respectively. This same dispersion relation occurs for waves in hot plasmas and transmission lines, which might form closed loops more similar to the periodic boundary condition appropriate for neocortical standing waves. If the springs are disconnected, only the global dynamics remain. Or, if the string tension is relaxed, only the local dynamics remain. Next we approach the behavior of the non-linear system described by the basic string equation, in which local and global effects are integrated.

The quantum model of the brain waves. The structure of the spectrum of the brain waves strongly depends on the state of the brain (Ecless, 1989). The illness of the brain is reflected in the spectrum of the waves. In physics, we can invent the mathematical models which help in the understanding of the processes. Take as an example: cosmic relic radiation (CRR). The spectrum of the CRR is well-analyzed with the help of the "black body" formula. However, nobody would imagine that somewhere, 10^{17} years ago, the Universe was a "black body." In this chapter, we develop the "black body" formula for the wave emission of the brain source (Marciak-Kozlowska and Kozlowski, 2006). We take as granted the empirical fact that electrodes detects and measure the weak electromagnetic waves, including *delta, theta, alpha, beta, gamma*, shown in Table 1. The waves have the prescribed frequencies in the range of Hz and amplitudes in the range of μV. In order to put forward the classical theory of the brain waves, Eq. (6) we will quantize the field Φ (x, t). In the model, we assume (i) the brain is the thermal source in local equilibrium with temperature T and (ii) the spectrum of the brain waves is quantized according to the formula

$$E = \hbar\omega \tag{8}$$

where E is the photon energy in eV, $\hbar$ =Planck constant, $\omega = 2\pi v, v$ -is the frequency in Hz. In Table 1, the frequencies and amplitudes are presented (Tuszyński, Dixon, 2002). We also assume that (iii) the number of photons emitted by the brain is proportional to the $(\text{amplitude})^2$ as for classical waves. The energies of the photons are the maximum values of energies of waves mentioned in Table 1. For the emission of black body brain waves, we propose the well know formula for the black body radiation

$$\frac{dN}{dE} = BE_{\max}^2 e^{(-\frac{E_{\max}}{T})} \tag{9}$$

where B is the normalization constant, B is the temperature of the brain thermal source, and the function $\frac{dN}{dE}$ describes the energy spectrum of the emitted brain photons. In Figure 2, the calculated energy spectrum, formula (9), is presented. In Figure 3, we present the result of the comparison of the calculated and observed spectra of the brain waves. The calculated spectra are normalized to the maximum of the measured spectra. The calculated spectra are for the temperature of the brain source T= 0.8 10^{-14} eV. The obtained temperature is the temperature for the brain source in the thermal equilibrium. The source, for an unknown reason, is thermally isolated (adiabatic well). However in very exceptional cases, the spectrum is changed by the tunneling to the quantum potential well. The temperature 1 eV ≅ 10^4 K relates, then, to the brain wave thermal spectra T=0.8 10^{-14} eV= 0.8 10^{-10} K. The calculated temperature of the brain source is much lower than CRR temperature= 2.7K.

Table 1. Spectrum of brain waves

Wave (Tuszyński, Dixon, 2002)	Range of frequencies (Hz)	Maximal values of frequencies (Hz)	Amplitude [μV]	Maximal values of energies (eV}	Amplitude^2
Delta	0, 5-4	4	100.0	7x 10^{-15}	10^4
Theta	4-8	8	110.0	1.7 x10^{-14}	1.2x 10^4
Alpha	8-13	13	40.0	3.4 x10^{-14}	1.6 x10^3
Beta	13-30	30	11.0	7 x10^{-14}	1.2x 10^2
Gamma	30-100	100	4.0	1.4 10^{-13}	16.0

It must be stressed that we abandon the idea that every physical object is either a wave or a particle. Neither it is possible to say that particles “become” waves in the quantum domain and, conversely, that waves are “transformed” into particles. It is therefore necessary to acknowledge that we have here a different kind of an entity – one that is specifically quantum. For this reason, Levy-Leblond and Balibar developed the name *quanton* (Levy-Leblond, Balibar, 1990). Following that idea, the human brain emits *quantons* with energies $E = \hbar\omega$ formula (8). The brain quantons are the quantum objects that follows all quantum laws: tunneling, superposition, and Heisenberg uncertainty rule. For if the wave length of the *quantons* were of the order of Earth’s radius, the quantum nature of the brain would be manifested in the Universe’s scale.

The above results present for the first time the *experimental neuroquantology*. The electromagnetic waves of the brain are analyzed in the framework of quantum mechanics. The classical electromagnetic waves emitted by the brain are quantized and the brain’s pulsations are presented as *quantons* with very small energies of the order of 10^{-15} to 10^{-13} eV. The result of our chapter is that the brain is a thermal source with temperatures in the range of

10^{-14} eV, i.e. 10^{-10} K. Considering that the human body temperature (and the brain) is equal to 309 K, it is hard to imagine that the emission of brain waves is the result of chemical reactions only. It seems that the Hameroff-Penrose suggestion that phenomena of consciousness are linked to the Planck Epoch help in understanding the results obtained in this chapter. The brain waves are linked to a very early time in the history of the Universe.

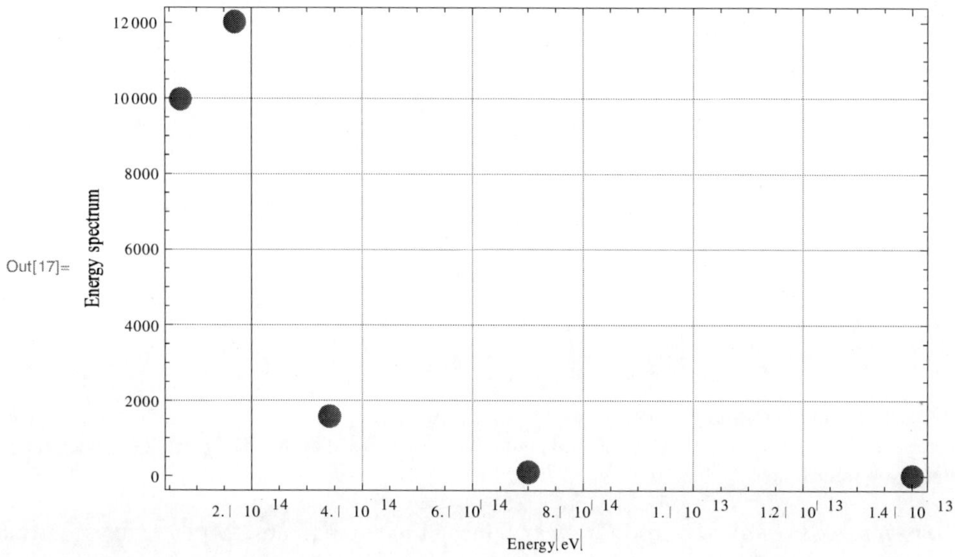

Figure 1. The energies of the photons are the maximum values of energies of waves mentioned.

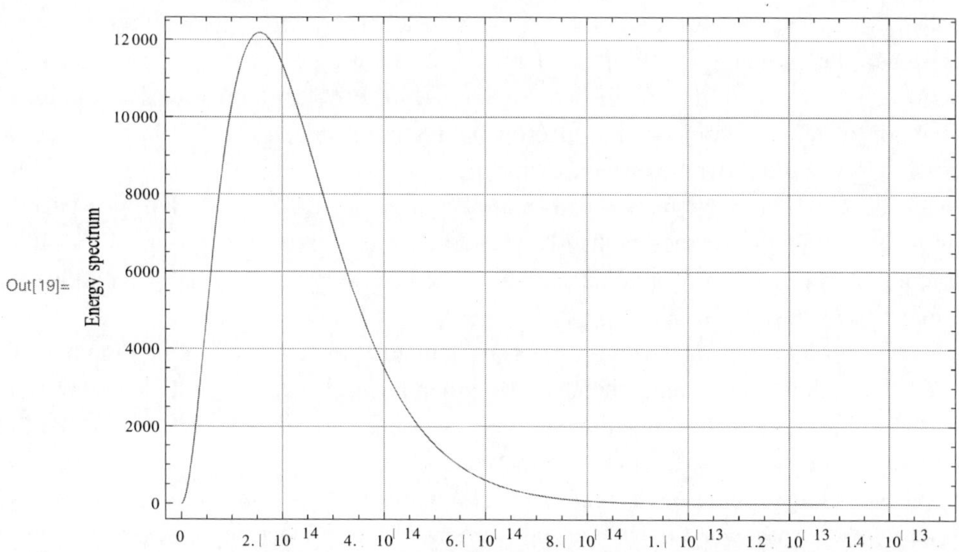

Figure 2. The calculated energy spectrum, formula (9) is presented.

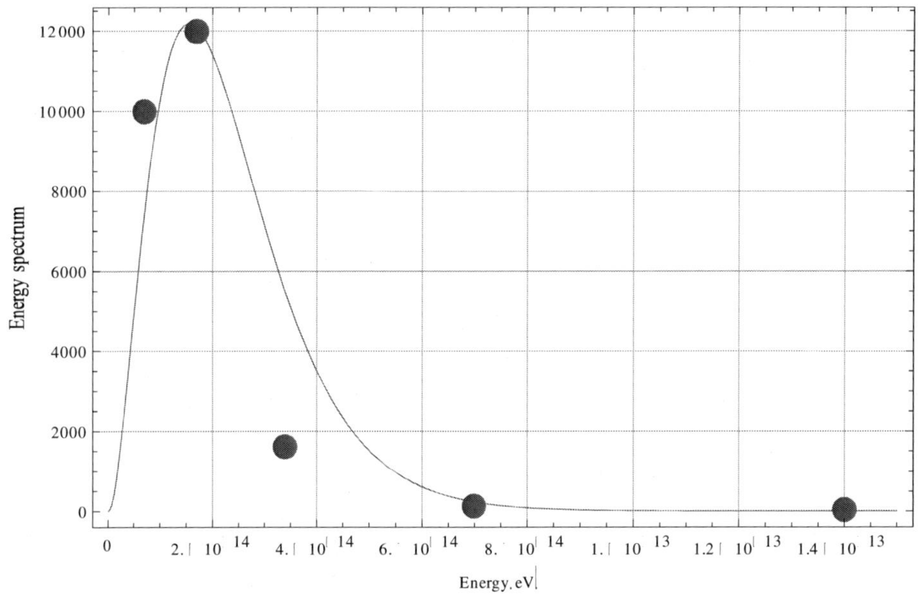

Figure 3. We present the result of the comparison of the calculated and observed spectra of the brain waves. The calculated spectra are normalized to the maximum of the measured spectra. The calculated spectra are for temperature of brain source T= 0.8 10^{-14} eV.

Consciousness=quantum string states? The ability of humans to perceive is currently going through a crucial change. More and more humans are able to notice fine-material energy fields and, thus, take up contact with other levels of our existence. This extended perception is sometimes enhanced through "Remote Viewing" techniques, forms of controlled extrasensory perception which were developed by the American military in the 1970s under the pseudonym "Project Stargate." It shows up that these remote viewing protocols – in the meantime, published to a large extent – not only make possible the investigation of far-away objects, but also opens a gate to hidden realities in our "here and now," which we could prove by own experiments.

With the same methods, human consciousness may move freely not only in space, but also in time. Through our experiments, we found that it is thereby even possible for humans to explore their own earlier incarnations and to exceed the limits of personal perception – also in cosmic dimensions!

Therefore, in place of the too-narrow term "Remote Viewing," we defined the new term "Refined Perception." It contains, thereby, not only a form of "seeing," but also other senses such as feeling, radiesthetic phenomena like dowsing, and above all in addition, the perception with the help of the human energy field, the aura.

The newest scientific research resulted in finding that humans can get into resonance with the earth and with other organisms via their different bodily electromagnetic fields. In this chapter, thereby, the electromagnetic waves produced by the human brain are our main field of interest.

The investigation of the earth resonance frequencies and/or the so-called Schumann waves is the key for the new scientific realizations. These are also well-known in esoteric circles, however usually presented in a physically-incorrect manner.

Nevertheless, Tesla Schumann waves will become already now increasingly important for all of us. The natural "magic chant" of the earth has a broad influence on our world climate and, in addition, on the evolution of human consciousness, and they have for a long time been the subject of doubtful military technologies. For a long time, we have known that the electrically positively-loaded ionosphere forms a pole with the negatively-charged earth's surface, and that between both an electrical tension constantly prevails. This tension unloads itself regularly, whenever a thunderstorm takes place somewhere. Such a system of two concentric, oppositely-charged balls in physics is called a ball condenser.

These physical characteristics of the ionosphere are used technically in the wireless information transfer. For radio waves, which are emitted from a transmitter on earth, the ionosphere works like an enormous hollow mirror. From this, the radio waves will be reflected and in such a way transferred over large distances.

Everyone who tried once to hear a far radio station with a medium wave radio knows the effect that the reception becomes obviously better after sunset. The reason is that the breakdown effects by the sun exposure to the ionosphere are then omitted.

These physical facts were described for the first time at the beginning of our century by the Croatian physicist and inventor Nikola Tesla, who accomplished at this time experiments for wireless transfer of energy at Colorado Springs.

Tesla produced at that time enormous electrical tensions of a hundred thousand volts with his experimental assemblies, with which he could produce even artificial lightning. He found out the fact that with every such lightning, radio waves of extremely low frequency are also radiated, which can penetrate through and into the earth almost without resistance. Thus, he had discovered the electromagnetic resonance frequency of the earth.

Tesla's work encountered at that time little approval, and because the economic use was not immediately foreseeable, his financial backers withdrew themselves rapidly, so that he could not complete his research work. Thus, it took nearly a half century, until someone else encountered this effect – a–gain, more or less by coincidence.

In the year 1952, the German physicist Professor Dr. W. O. Schumann of the Technical University of Munich wanted to give his students exercises regarding the physics of electricity. At that time, he worked with them on the computation of ball condensers. In order not to let it become too theoretical and abstract, Professor Schumann said to his students: "Imagine the ionosphere as the one ball and the earth's surface as the other ball. Calculate then, what will be the results." Schumann had no idea which value would result from this, and to be able to examine his students' work, he took a pencil and a sheet of paper and made a rough calculation. He found a value of approximately 10 Hz (Schumann, 1952).

To illustrate, this value is the resonance frequency of the earth, thus the frequency with which the earth begins to swing. Each energy discharge between the ionosphere and the earth's surface, thus each normal thunderbolt, produces radio waves of such a frequency, which are in resonance with the earth as a by-product. They cannot, therefore, merely penetrate into the earth, but at the same time accumulate whereby it comes to the formation of enormous standing waves, which may remain stable over long time.

Schumann himself at that time in no way knew about the consequences of his discovery. Nevertheless, he published the result in a physical technical periodical. After that, the Schumann frequency, as it is called today in honor of its discovery, would probably land in the waste-paper basket of science history, but a physically-interested physician coincidentally read the paper. He called to Schumann immediately because the physician was extremely excited about what he read there. The Schumann frequency is also the resonance frequency of the human brain!

Measurements of the brain waves of humans with an electrical encephalograph show that the brain produces electromagnetic waves, which lie in the range between 1 and 40 Hz. This spectrum is in medicine divided into four ranges, which accompany different consciousness conditions:

1. Delta waves (1-3 Hz) are characteristic of dreamless deep sleep and coma conditions.
2. Theta waves (4-7 Hz) are characteristic of dream sleep.
3. Alpha waves (8-12 Hz) arise in the relaxed awake condition, e. g. in a meditation or briefly before falling asleep and/or immediately after awaking.
4. Beta waves (13-40 Hz) are dominant in the normal awake condition.

The physician explained to Schumann that it was nevertheless a strange coincidence that the earth and brain have homogeneous resonance frequencies, and so Schumann instructed his graduate student and later successor to his chair, Herbert Konig, to further investigate this. Konig, who also became well-known for his scientific investigations about the dowsing phenomenon some years ago, accomplished, in the context of his doctoral work, extensive measurements of the earth's resonance frequency and, thereby, naturally came to a more exact value than Schumann during his rough calculation. The accurate value of the Schumann frequency is 7.83 Hz.

Thus, it is finally clear that the agreement with the human brain frequencies is not coincidental, because this value corresponds accurately to the fundamental brain frequency of most mammals. For humans, it lies scarcely at the lower limit of the alpha range, thus at the border between sleep and being awake. Is this the reason that animals have a less-evolved consciousness compared with man? Are they only at the threshold of higher consciousness?

The agreement between earth and brain frequency is indeed no coincidence because animals and humans are children of the earth and their brain frequencies adapted quite easily to the natural conditions of their habitat in the process of the evolution.

It is well known in science that the brain reacts to electromagnetic frequencies which are offered to it from the outside if they are in the correct frequency range. This is a typical resonance effect. Many of the 'mind machines' are based on this principle, which should be helpful to achieve a relaxed, meditative condition, thus the alpha condition, where the calm waves of 8-12 Hz dominate and the restless thought activities of the normal beta condition cease. Now, the lowest classical 7.83 Hz frequency is without any doubt the most intensive, but the higher form of a spectrum of different oscillations, to which the brain is altogether sensitive. The Schumann frequency spectrum is remarkably similar to that of the human brain, because, similarly in EEG measurements, the alpha and theta frequencies are characterized by far, high excursions, while the beta waves are flat and jerky. Thus, the Schumann waves as a whole tend rather to calm down and wake up the human brain at the same time. The result might be a condition of brain synchronization, which is momentarily still difficult to conceive for us. The newest results in brain research show that the old conception was too naive and that the brain simply reconstructs available frequencies from the outside, meaning that the conception does not describe the real procedures. Instead, the brain reacts to outside energies and oscillations to which it is sensitive, with an extensive reorganization of its internal circuits. This leads – similar to the decrease of the magnetic field – to a chaotic, stress-promoting unrest effect. Then, however, the brain is inclined to organize itself on a higher oscillation level again. It achieves a higher consciousness condition, which is not explainable from the sum of the two single conditions.

This condition of how it is reached by meditation techniques like the tables of Chartres or certain tape cartridges cannot only be described as brain synchronization. This higher consciousness condition is somewhat more powerful. Perhaps one can describe it best as a condition in which humans are awake and asleep at the same time, and the normal daily consciousness with the ability for critical, free decision and the immeasurable possibilities of the subconsciousness are available at the same time. In this condition, human consciousness transcends the fourth dimension – man becomes the master of time. There is, at least in our culture, presently only one consciousness condition in which this is realized – the so-called lucid dream. Normally, awake consciousness is more or less switched off during a typical dream, which is also recognizable by the fact that in the dream condition, the theta and alpha waves dominate. Humans are therefore predominantly passive in their dreams and let the dream action evolve itself.

Critical abilities are to a large extent suppressed in dreams, so that the bizarre realities, which one meets usually in dreams, are not noticed during the dream. This essentially corresponds to the consciousness condition of "dream time" in former times, in which humans were more or less delivered to external influences in their daily life and were able only to react. They could nevertheless survive – similar to the animals – since they were an integrated part of the total structure of nature. Quite simply, the consciousness of the free will, which could enable them to revolt, was missing to them. In daily consciousness, our rational understanding dominates, which lets us meet critical and self-conscious decisions. On the other hand, the immeasurable creative forces of the unconscious are now in the background – forces which permit us to create whole realities in our dreams. Also, this limits our scope of action because our awake understanding is not able to seize and control nature in its entirety. Our rational understanding is inclined to define itself, and so, in the wisdom of the unconscious, the feeling of belonging to a larger entireness is missing. In the condition of the lucid dream, these two contrasts are bridged. One becomes conscious during the dream of the fact that one dreams, and so one knows that the reality is experienced was created totally by the dreamer. The creative forces of the unconscious are fully at his disposal. On the other hand, his critical understanding is also active, so that his ability to engage in self-conscious acting is available as well.

Thus, the lowest Schumann frequency is not today already any longer with those 7.83 Hz, *g* in the fifties, but over far distances of the year already in the proximity of the "magical" border of 8 Hz, sometimes even higher. We called this border "magical" because it represents exactly the transition from the theta to the alpha frequencies. Only in such moments it be will possible to let the consciousness-extending effect of the Schumann resonance spectrum as a whole become fully effective because the sleep-inducing, i.e. consciousness-clouding effect of the theta waves is void. The highest frequency values occur thereby in the summer months (of the Northern Hemisphere), while they drop down again in winter. The trend is still confirmed by investigations of the second and third Schumann resonance frequencies. Here, the seasonal fluctuations are to be observed even more strongly. They move between 13.8 and 14.1 Hz and between 19.5 and 20.3 Hz.

What does this mean for our consciousness? Research over unusual consciousness conditions, as, for instance, the psychologist Michael Murphy performed, points out that shamans or Indian fakirs reach the most pronounced metanormal abilities in conditions which one cannot describe with the usual term "trance," which is what we mostly understand as a sleep-similar condition of lowered consciousness. Rather, it concerns a feeling of increased awakeness, thus a condition of the excitation or ecstasy that is characterized in the EEG rather by the higher beta frequencies above 20 Hz (Chand, 2009).

If, due to the climatic changes on earth, the natural spectrum of the Schumann waves would thus constantly expose us, on the one hand, with intensifying alpha frequency, and, on the other hand, however, a simultaneous ever-intensifying beta wave spectrum, which is appropriate to a large extent above 20 Hz, then this would mean that we are all going towards a condition of increased awakeness. This is strengthened still, as we see, by the continuous decrease of the earth's magnetic field.

If we see, however, these effects as a whole, then we will feel this consciousness condition no longer as stress or we will become sick. The reassuring alpha waves take care of this, which have the largest intensity in the Schumann wave spectrum. Rather, it might be a very balanced, positive consciousness condition. Since it does not concern a pure alpha condition, we will not be in danger of increased manipulations. Everything indicates that, regardless of all global dangers, mankind steers on a new age of higher consciousness, not from own drive, but steered by the "charm singing" of the earth. Were the old prophecies wrong? On the contrary, we will see that 2000 year old writings already foresaw this development accurately!

Can a quantum effect be seen? The plain answer is no, of course. By definition, quantum superpositions are what exist prior to measurement. As soon as a measurement is made, the rules dictate that one particular result out of the range of possible results must be obtained, so that the simultaneous presence of two different states can never be directly demonstrated. As always, the mysterious, inscrutable parts of quantum mechanics remain hidden from our eyes (which is why they are mysterious and inscrutable: if quantum superpositions were to be found in the world of our senses, we would long ago have developed a language for them, and would not find them unfamiliar).

We can, nevertheless, see the effects or consequences of quantum superpositions. The two-slit experiment remains the prime example: a single photon somehow passing through a two-slit apparatus creates an interference pattern in a way that a strictly locatable classical particle could not possibly do. If you insist on saying, in particle language, that the photon must go through one slit or the other, you cannot understand the interference pattern, which in wave terms requires that some contribution comes from each slit. It is only by accepting the idea of the superposition of states, in which there are coexisting pieces of wave function describing photons that go through both slits, that you can begin to understand how interference in such a case can happen. But at the same time, you have to be wary of imagining that the parts of the wave function associated with each slit have anything to do with actual photons going through actual slits—things get tricky, as we have seen, as soon as you start imputing a traditional degree of reality to these equipresent bits and pieces of wavefunction.

These familiar examples of superposition—the two-slit experiment, electrons prior to spin measurement, or photons prior to a polarization measurement—apply to single objects, individual quantum creatures. Can large systems—ones composed of lots of photons, electron, or atoms—behave in the same way? Not easily, it turns out, but there is at least one reputable and instructive example.

The example comes from certain kinds of superconducting devices, which, when cooled to suitably-low temperatures, conduct electricity without any resistance. An electric current set up in a ring of superconducting material will flow around and around forever, without loss. Because of resistance, an electric current set up in a ring of copper wire, for example, will come to a halt almost the instant the motive power is turned off.

This is not the place to discuss in any detail the complex and demanding theory of superconductivity, which was not put together until almost half a century after the phenomenon itself was first discovered, back in 1911. All we need to know here is that the electrons in a superconductor move in a coherent fashion. In both an ordinary copper wire and a superconductor, electric current amounts to a collective flow of electrons, but in a copper wire, the electrons jostle about like a huge crowd trying to follow a parade down narrow streets. They bump up against the copper atoms of the wire and each other, and the incessant jostling and obstructing and diversion amount to a resistance to the flow. It takes effort—in the form of a voltage applied to the wire—to keep all the electrons moving along.

But in a superconductor, the electrons abandon all sense of individual identity and purpose, and move as one. It is not that every electron is doing the same thing as every other electron, but that they all move in a coherent fashion. A human example of such coherence is the wave that crowds perform at a baseball game. If everyone in the stadium stands up and sits down at random, all you'll see is confusion, but when everyone harmonizes their motion, a wave appears to travel around the stands. An interesting phenomenon occurs here: as one person at one place in the crowd is standing up, another person, perhaps on the opposite side of the stadium, is sitting down. As the wave moves around, you could spot any number of such pairs of people whose up-and-down motions are exactly harmonized. The electrons in a superconductor behave something like this. They link up in pairs, not in the sense of being physically linked, but in the sense that their motions are coupled even though the electrons are a long way apart.

In terms of quantum mechanics, the upshot of this harmony is that all electron pairs in a superconductor are described by the same wave function (all the pairs of people in the baseball doing the same thing), as conducting ring, in which something else happens: because all the electron pairs follow a single wave function, that wave function has to wrap around on itself in the ring without any abrupt change. Among the implications of this wave function continuity is that any magnetic field passing through the interior loop, connected as it is to the current flowing around the loop, becomes "quantized," meaning that it can take on only certain discrete values.

It is not too difficult these days to make a superconducting ring centimeters or more across, and yet even this large an object should, if quantum theory is correct, be correctly described as a single quantum system characterized by the current flowing through it and the magnetic field trapped inside it. Even though it is a large, compound object with an electric current and magnetic field that arise from the motion of countless electrons, it is, or should be, a single quantum system, just as an individual electron or photon is a single quantum object.

An unbroken ring, once set up, will carry current forever. It remains, in other words, in a fixed quantum state. A more interesting state of affairs can be created by putting a small gap somewhere in the ring, so that the electrical circuit is not quite a full circle but has a slightly resistive "weak link" somewhere along its circumference. As long as the gap is narrow, the superconducting current will continue to flow, being able in effect to jump across the gap. But the presence of the gap allows, roughly-speaking, the magnetic field threading the ring to come and go a little; it is no longer strictly-confined, and additional increments of the magnetic field can jump into the ring through the gap, or out of it the same way. Now we have a quantum system, characterized by a certain intensity of magnetic field, which can jump from one state to another.

Difficult and elaborate experiments have been performed in the last few years in which the imposition of an external magnetic field is used to control the stability of the individual quantum states of the ring, and to influence the ease with which it can jump from one state to another. The system does indeed jump in the manner prescribed by quantum mechanics, and certain sophisticated results can be obtained which indicate magnetic field can exist in a genuinely superposed state the simultaneous presence of different magnetic states of the ring.

Of course, these superpositions, as we said at the outset, cannot directly demonstrated, because any measurement of the magnetic state forces it to adopt one specific value or another. Rather, certain measurements of other properties of the ring which do not interfere with its magnetic state are consistent with the existence of a superposition of magnetic states the ring.

In short, everything works the way quantum mechanics says they work. What does this tell us? Mainly, that in this respect, it is possible to have a macroscopic system that follows the rules of quantum mechanics. That is an important fact, because it had been thought from time to time that the way of escaping the measurement problem would be to create macroscopic systems, as opposed to individual quanta, which would not obey the elementary rules of quantum states, and so could not sustain superposed states. The inducting ring is a counterexample to that hypothesis: it is definitely a macroscopic system, but it evidently behaves just as quantum theory predicts. You cannot get around the measurement problem by supposing that, for some reason, large objects and systems obey a different set of rules.

One might say that the traditional two-slit experiment is an optic demonstration of the correctness of quantum mechanics since one ends up with a large apparatus and a result—the appearance of an interference pattern—that's easily visible to the naked eye. But in the two-slit experiment, the fundamental quantum object is the individual photon going through the apparatus, whereas in the superconducting ring, the quantum states represent collective motions of trillions of individual electrons pair acting together.

In short, it is not the case that just putting together a lot of individual quantum objects necessarily erases quantum behavior. On the other hand, a superconductor is an exquisitely special and unusual creation, and electrons in large systems generally do not get along so well together. If it's true that superconductors exhibit large-scale quantum behavior only because of the very special conditions under which they exist, then perhaps we should ask in what way ordinary, non-superconducting systems are different, and if that difference has anything to do with why, for the most part, they do not apparently show quantum behavior.

Modified Schrödinger Equation. In a paper, Kozlowski and Marciak-Kozlowski (2010) proposed new Schrodinger equations for the brain:

$$i\hbar\frac{\partial\Psi}{\partial t}=-\frac{\hbar^2}{2m_i}\nabla^2\Psi+V\Psi-\frac{\hbar^2}{2M_p}\nabla^2\Psi$$
$$+\frac{\hbar^2}{2M_p}\nabla^2\Psi-\frac{\hbar^2}{2M_pc^2}\frac{\partial^2\Psi}{\partial t^2}. \tag{1}$$

In formula (1) M_p is the mass Planck, m_i is the mass of the particle. In the paper (Kozlowski, Marciak-Kozlowska, 2010), the new interpretation of the equation (1) was discovered. We argue that the $\Psi(x,y,z,t)$ represents the state of consciousness, presumably the Bohm function, which fulfils the wave equation

$$\frac{\hbar^2}{2M_p}\nabla^2\Psi-\frac{\hbar^2}{2M_pc^2}\frac{\partial^2\Psi}{\partial t^2}=0, \tag{2}$$

i.e. $\Psi(x,y,z,t)$ is the Bohm pilot wave. For $M_p\neq 0$ Eq. (2) can be written as

$$\nabla^2\Psi-\frac{1}{c^2}\frac{\partial^2\Psi}{\partial t^2}=0. \tag{3}$$

It is interesting to observe that pilot brain wave Ψ does not depend on the mass of the particle. With postulate (3), we obtain from equation (1)

$$i\hbar\frac{\partial\Psi}{\partial t}=-\frac{\hbar^2}{2m_i}\nabla^2\Psi+V\Psi-\frac{\hbar^2}{2M_p}\nabla^2\Psi \tag{4}$$

and simultaneously

$$\frac{\hbar^2}{2M_p}\nabla^2\Psi-\frac{\hbar^2}{2M_pc^2}\frac{\partial^2\Psi}{\partial t^2}=0. \tag{5}$$

In the operator form Eq. (5) can be written as

$$\hat{E} = \frac{\hat{p}^2}{2m_i} + \frac{1}{2M_p c^2}\hat{E}^2, \tag{6}$$

where $\hat{E}$ and $\hat{p}$ denote the operators for energy and momentum of the particle with mass m_i. Equation (31) is the new dispersion relation for quantum particle with mass m_i. From Eq. (21) one can conclude that Schrödinger quantum mechanics is valid for particles with mass $m_i \ll M_P$. But a pilot wave exists independent of the mass of the particles.

For particles with mass $m_i \ll M_P$ Eq. (5) has the form

$$i\hbar\frac{\partial\Psi}{\partial t} = -\frac{\hbar^2}{2m_i}\nabla^2\Psi + V\Psi. \tag{7}$$

Equation (8) is the standard Schrodinger equation for quantum phenomena.

In the case when $m_i \approx M_p$ Eq. (5) can be written as

$$i\hbar\frac{\partial\Psi}{\partial t} = -\frac{\hbar^2}{2M_p}\nabla^2\Psi + V\Psi, \tag{8}$$

but considering Eq. (4) one obtains

$$i\hbar\frac{\partial\Psi}{\partial t} = -\frac{\hbar^2}{2M_p c^2}\frac{\partial^2\Psi}{\partial t^2} + V\Psi \tag{9}$$

or

$$\frac{\hbar^2}{2M_p c^2}\frac{\partial^2\Psi}{\partial t^2} + i\hbar\frac{\partial\Psi}{\partial t} - V\Psi = 0. \tag{10}$$

Gravity and Schrödinger Equation: Tesla-Schumann waves. Recently, there has been growing interest in the Tesla-Schumann resonances. It is well-known that the frequencies of the Tesla-Schumann resonances have the same values as the human brain waves. In this section, we will discuss the influence of the gravity on the function $\Psi(x, y, z, t)$

Classically, when the inertial mass m_i and the gravitational mass m_g are equated, the mass drops out of Newton's equation of motion, implying that particles of different mass with the same initial conditions follows the same trajectories. But in Schrödinger's equation, the masses do not cancel. For example, in a uniform gravitational field

$$i\hbar\frac{\partial\Psi}{\partial t}=-\frac{\hbar^2}{2m_i}\frac{\partial^2\Psi}{\partial x^2}+m_g gx\Psi \tag{11}$$

g=gravity acceleration (12)

implying mass dependent difference in motion.

In this section, we investigate the motion of a particle with inertial mass m_i in the potential field V. The potential V contains all the possible interactions, including the gravity.

$$i\hbar\frac{\partial\Psi}{\partial t}=V\Psi-\frac{\hbar^2}{2m_i}\nabla^2\Psi-2\tau\hbar\frac{\partial^2\Psi}{\partial t^2} \tag{13}$$

where the term

$$2\tau\hbar\frac{\partial^2\Psi}{\partial t^2},$$

with

$$\tau=\frac{\hbar}{m_i v^2} \tag{14}$$

describes the memory of the particle with mass m_i. The above equation for the wave function Ψ is the local equation with finite invariant speed, c which equals the light speed in the vacuum.

Let us look for the solution of the Eq. (13), V=0, in the form (for 1D)

$$\Psi=\Psi(x-ct). \tag{15}$$

For $\tau\neq 0$, i.e. for finite Planck mass we obtain:

$$\Psi(x-ct)=\exp\left(\frac{2\mu ic}{\hbar}(x-ct)\right) \tag{16}$$

where the reduced μ mass equals

$$\mu=\frac{m_i M_p}{m_i+M_p} \tag{17}$$

For $m_i << M_p$, i.e. for all elementary particles one obtains

$$\mu=m_i \tag{18}$$

and formula (16) describes the wave function for free Schrödinger particles

$$\Psi(x-ct)=\exp\left(\frac{2m_i ic}{\hbar}(x-ct)\right) \tag{19}$$

For $m_i >> M_p$, $\mu = M_p$

$$\Psi(x-ct)=\exp\left(\frac{2M_p ic}{\hbar}(x-ct)\right) \tag{20}$$

From formula (19), we conclude that $\Psi(x-ct)$ is independent of mass m_i. In the case $m_i < M_p$ from formulae (19) and (20), one obtains

$$\mu = m_i\left(1-\frac{m_i}{M_p}\right)$$

$$\Psi(x-ct)=\exp\left(\frac{2im_i c}{\hbar}(x-ct)\right)\exp\left(-i\frac{m_i}{M_p}\left(\frac{2m_i c}{\hbar}x-\frac{2m_i c^2}{\hbar}t\right)\right) \tag{21}$$

In formula (21) we put

$$k=\frac{2m_i c}{\hbar}$$

$$\omega=\frac{2m_i c^2}{\hbar}$$

and obtain

$$\Psi(x-ct)=e^{i(kx-\omega t)}e^{-i\frac{m_i}{M_p}(kx-\omega t)} \tag{22}$$

As can be concluded from formula (22), the second term depends on the gravity

$$\exp\left[-i\frac{m_i}{M_p}(kx-\omega t)\right]=\exp\left[-i\left(\frac{m_i^2 G}{\hbar c}\right)^{½}(kx-\omega t)\right] \tag{23}$$

where G is the Newton gravity constant. Formula (22) describes the influence of the gravity on the state of the consciousness.

It is interesting to observe that the new constant, α_G,

$$\alpha_G = \frac{m_i^2 G}{\hbar c} \tag{24}$$

is the gravitational constant. For $m_i = m_N$ nucleon mass

$$\alpha_G = 5.9042 \cdot 10^{-39} \tag{25}$$

The Particle in a Box

In a forthcoming paper, we propose the quantum model of the consciousness waves. We show that instead of waves *alpha, beta, theta, delta, gamma*, we can speak about *quantons alpha, beta, gamma, delta, theta.* In this section, we consider the simplest model for the emission of quantons.

We consider quantum mechanical system for a particle of mass m_i confined in a one-dimensional box of length *L and with infinite walls*. For the particle to be confined within region II, the potential energy outside (regions I and III) is assumed to be infinite. In order to understand this system further, we need to formulate and solve the Schrödinger equations (26).

$$i\hbar\frac{\partial \Psi}{\partial t} = -\frac{\hbar^2}{2m_i}\nabla^2\Psi + V\Psi - \frac{\hbar^2}{2M_p}\nabla^2\Psi + \frac{\hbar^2}{2M_p}\left(\nabla^2\Psi - \frac{1}{c^2}\frac{\partial^2\Psi}{\partial t^2}\right). \tag{26}$$

Considering the pilot wave equation

$$\nabla^2\Psi - \frac{1}{c^2}\frac{\partial^2\Psi}{\partial t^2} = 0 \tag{27}$$

one obtains

$$i\hbar\frac{\partial \Psi}{\partial t} = -\frac{\hbar^2}{2\mu}\nabla^2\Psi + V\Psi, \tag{28}$$

where

$$\mu = \frac{m_i M_p}{m_i + M_p}.$$

In region II, $V(x)=0$	In regions I and III, $V(x)=\infty$
$-\frac{\hbar^2}{2\mu}\nabla^2\Psi+V\Psi=E\Psi$	$-\frac{\hbar^2}{2\mu}\nabla^2\Psi+V\Psi=E\Psi$
$-\frac{\hbar^2}{2\mu}\nabla^2\Psi+0=E\Psi$	$-\frac{\hbar^2}{2\mu}\nabla^2\Psi+\infty\Psi=E\Psi$
$-\frac{\hbar^2}{2\mu}\nabla^2\Psi=E\Psi$	$-\frac{\hbar^2}{2\mu}\nabla^2\Psi=(E-\infty)\Psi$

For regions I and III (outside the box), the solution is straightforward, the wavefunction Ψ is zero. For region II (inside the box), we need to find a function that regenerates itself after taking its second derivative.

$$-\frac{\hbar^2}{2\mu}\nabla^2\Psi=E\Psi$$

$$\nabla^2\Psi=\frac{2\mu E}{\hbar^2}\Psi=-k^2\Psi, \quad \text{where we define } k=\sqrt{\frac{2\mu E}{\hbar^2}}. \tag{29}$$

Perfect candidates would be the trigonometric sine and cosine functions.

$$\Psi(x)=A\cos(kx)+B\sin(kx). \tag{30}$$

To further refine the wave function, we need to impose boundary conditions: At *x=0*, the wave function should be zero.

$$\Psi(0)=A\cos(k0)+B\sin(k0)=A\cdot 1+B\cdot 0. \tag{31}$$

Equation can only be true if $A = 0$: $\Psi(x)=B\sin(kx)$.

In addition, at *x=L*, the wave function should also be zero.

$$\Psi(0)=0=B\sin(kL). \quad \text{True when } kL=n\pi \text{ or } k=\frac{n\pi}{L}:$$

$$\Psi(x)=B\sin(\frac{n\pi}{L}x), \quad n=1,2,3,... \tag{32}$$

Going back to the Schrödinger's equation, we can then formulate the energies

$$kL = n\pi \quad \text{and} \quad k = \sqrt{\frac{2\mu E}{\hbar^2}}$$

$$\sqrt{\frac{2\mu E}{\hbar^2}} = \frac{n\pi}{L} \Rightarrow \frac{2\mu E}{\hbar^2} = \frac{n^2\pi^2}{L^2}$$

$$E_n = \frac{n^2\pi^2\hbar^2}{2\mu L^2} = \frac{n^2h^2}{8\mu L^2} \quad \text{since } \hbar = \frac{h}{2\pi}. \tag{34}$$

Thus, the application of the Schrödinger equation to this problem results in the well-known expressions for the wave functions and energies, namely:

$$\Psi_n = \sqrt{\frac{2}{L}}\sin\left(\frac{n\pi x}{L}\right) \quad \text{and} \quad E_n = \frac{n^2h^2}{8\mu L^2}. \tag{35}$$

From formula (60) we conclude that for "heavy" classical particles, i.e. for $m_i >> M_p$ the energy spectrum of the particle in the box is independent of the mass of particle

$$E_n = \frac{n^2h^2}{8M_pL^2}. \tag{36}$$

In a paper (Marciak-Kozłowska, Kozłowski, 2010), we argue that formula (36) describes the quantum states of the consciousness. The energy of the quanta of the consciousness is of the order of 10^{-15} eV. Substituting 10^{-15} *eV* for E_n to formula (16) and considering the mass of $M_p = 10^{31}$ *eV* we obtain for the characteristic length, *L*, the value 10^{-6} nm., i.e. lower that the *nanotubule.* With $L=10^{-6}$ nm we obtain from formula (36) the following spectrum for brain waves

$$E_n - E_0 = 7x10^{-15}, 2.8x10^{-15}, 6.3x10^{-14}, 1.1x10^{-13}, 1.7x10^{-13} eV \tag{37}$$

for n=1, 2, 3, 3, 5 respectively.

The brain photons are emitted as quantum de-excitation in the quantum well, i.e. $\omega_n = \frac{E_n - E_0}{\hbar}$ where ω_n is the angular frequency of the brain photons with quantum number *n* and $E_n.E_0$ are the n-excited state for *n=1, 2, 3, 4, 5* respectively, and E_0 is ground state of the quantum well with energy equals zero. In Table 2, the comparison of the measured (EEG) and calculated spectra are presented. The agreement is rather good.

Table 2. Comparison of the measured (EEG) and calculated brain photons spectra

Measured energies, EEG (eV)	Model calculation EEG (eV)
7×10^{-15}	7×10^{-15}
1.7×10^{-14}	2.8×10^{-14}
3.4×10^{-14}	6.3×10^{-14}
7.0×10^{-14}	1.1×10^{-13}
1.4 x10-^{13}	1.7×10^{-13}

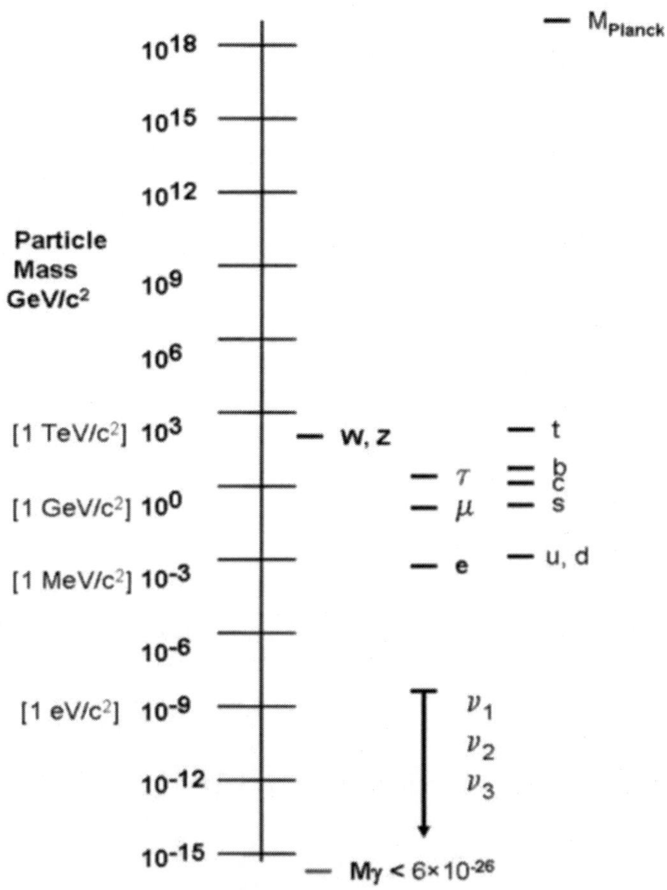

Figure 4. Energy 10^{-15} eV= Energy of the brain quantons.

In this paragraph we put forward the quantization of the brain waves. We propose the theoretical model: the well with infinite walls for the calculations of the brain photons (*quantons*) spectra. The model is free of additional parameters. By comparison to the measured EEG spectra, we obtain the width (dimension of the well) $L=10^{-6}$ *nm*. With value of *L*, we can calculate the whole spectrum of the brain pulsation. It is well known that frequencies ν (energies $\hbar\omega$) of the brain photons are nearly equal to the frequencies of the Tesla-Schumann waves, which are the resonances in the Earth-ionosphere cavity. In the paper, we investigate the influence of the gravitation on the brain pulsations and obtain the wave functions for gravity-dependent brain waves. The connections of the lighting, the Tesla-Schumann resonances, and brain waves can be supported by the observation that the primordial charge channel for lighting has the thickness of the order of 10^{-6} nm is of the order of the radius of atomic nucleus.

The calculations of the brain wave frequencies are based on the existence of the strand of the medium – the strand of the 10^{19} protons with width of the order of 10-15 m and length of the 10^{4}km – the string of the consciousness. The vibration of this string produces the brain waves. The energies of the brain waves are the energies of the standing waves of the consciousness string.

Could quantum physics speed-up biological evolution? The idea starts from the question how a complex protein or strand of DNA could possibly have formed by random trials and mere chance from primordial amino acids or a series of nucleotides up to the high degree of complexity that is required to drive self-replication and evolution. It has therefore been asked whether a faster, macroscopic quantum-sorting mechanism might have been involved in finding the first successfully self-replicating molecule on Earth (McFadden, 2000). However, its realization on our early Earth must have involved thousands of atoms and molecules in a warm and wet environment under the additional precondition that all sorts of molecules were available, that the formation of the sample molecular structures was energetically-accessible and that the molecules were delocalized over large areas in the given environment.

In particular, the latter requirement is in variance with the findings of molecule decoherence experiments (Hornberger et al., 2003), which confirm that any measurement – be it collision with other molecules, phonons, or photons – is capable of destroying the quantum delocalization if the interaction retrieves position information. But even if we hypothesize that large molecules could be delocalized in a primordial soup, the fastest speed-up in Grover's quantum search has still only a square-root advantage and the number of combinations is still stupendous. One might argue that the initial replicators were extremely tiny and that the first useful molecules for life were only influenced or catalyzed by the replication of the tinier structures. But even then, a feedback loop between biological evolution and the suggested quantum coherence remains highly speculative in the light of present knowledge.

References

Abbot, D, Davies, PC, and Pati, AK (2008). *Quantum aspects of life*. Imperial College Press.

Amico, L, Fazio, R, Osterloh, A, and Vedral, V (2008). Entanglement in many-body systems. *Rev. Mod. Phys.*, 80, 517–576.

Anderson, P (1958). Absence of diffusion in certain random lattices. *Phys. Rev.,* 109, 1492–1505.

Arieli, A., Shoham, D., Hildesheim, R. and Grinvald, A. Coherent spatiotemporal patterns of ongoing activity revealed by rela time optical imaging coupled with single –unit recording in the cat visual cortex, *J. Neurophys*., 1995, 73, 2072-2093.

Arndt, M, Nairz, O, Voss-Andreae, J, Keller, C, der Zouw, GV, and Zeilinger, A (1999). Wave-particle duality of C60 molecules. *Nature*, 401, 680–682.

Balabin, I and Onuchic, J (2000). Dynamically controlled protein tunneling paths in photosynthetic reaction centers. *Science*, 290, 114–117.

Balasubramanian, G, Chan, I, Kolesov, R, Al-Hmoud, M, Tisler, J, Shin, C, Kim, C, Wojcik, A, Hemmer, P, Krueger, A, Hanke, T, Leitenstorfer, A, Bratschitsch, R, Jelezko1, F, and Wrachtrup, J (2008). Nanoscale imaging magnetometry with diamond spins under ambient conditions. *Nature*, 455, 648–651.

Blankenship, RE (1989). Special issue - tunneling processes in photosynthesis. *Photosynthesis Research*, 22, 1-1.

Blankenship, RE (2002). *Molecular mechanisms of photosynthesis*. Blackwell Publishing, Oxford.

Bouwmeester, D, Ekert, A, and Zeilinger, A, editors (2000). *The physics of quantum information*. Springer-Verlag Berlin Heidelberg.

Brixner, T, Stenger, J, Vaswani, H, Cho, M, Blankenship, RE, and Fleming, G (2005). Two-dimensional spectroscopy of electronic couplings in photosynthesis. *Nature*, 434, 625–628.

Brookes, JC, Hartoutsiou, F, Horsfield, AP, and Stoneham, AM (2007). Could humans recognize odor by phonon assisted tunneling?. *Phys. Rev. Lett.*, 98(038101).

Brougham, DF, Caciuffo, R, and Horsewill, AJ (1999). Coordinated proton tunnelling in a cyclic network of four hydrogen bonds in the solid state. *Nature*, 397, 241–243.

Brukner, C, Vedral, V, and Zeilinger, A (2006). Crucial role of quantum entanglement in bulk properties of solids. *Phys. Rev. A*, 73(012110).

Buck, L and Axel, R (1991). A novel multigene family may encode odorant receptors - A molecular basis for odor recognition. *Cell*, 65, 175–187.

Cai, J, Guerreschi, GG, and Briegel, HJ (2009). *Quantum control and entanglement in a chemical compass*. arXiv:0906.2383.

Cai, J, Popescu, S, and Briegel, HJ (2008). *Dynamic entanglement in oscillating molecules*. arXiv:0809.4906v1.

Caruso, F, Chin, A, Datta, A, Huelga, S, and Plenio, M (2009). *Fundamental mechanisms of noise supported energy transfer in biological systems*. arXiv:0901.4454.

Cha, Y, Murray, C, and Klinman, J (1989). Hydrogen tunneling in enzyme reactions. *Science*, 243, 1325–1330.

Chand N, Israil M, Rai. J.Schuman resonance frequency variations observed in magnetotelluric data recorded from Garhwal Himalayan region India, *Ann. Geophys.*, 23, 3497-3507, 2009

Cheng, YC and Fleming, GR (2009). Dynamics of light harvesting in photosynthesis. *Annu. Rev. Phys. Chem.*, 60, 241–262.

Clauser, J (1997). De Broglie-wave interference of small rocks and live viruses. In Cohen, R, Horne, M, and Stachel, J, editors, *Experimental Metaphysics*, pages 1–11. Kluwer Academic.

Closs, GL (1969). Mechanism explaining nuclear spin polarizations in radical combination reactions. *J. Am. Chem. Soc.*, 91, 4552–4554.

Collini, E and Scholes, GD (2009). Coherent intrachain energy migration in a conjugated polymer at room temperature. *Science*, 323, 369 – 373.

Cory, DG, Price, MD, Maas, W, Knill, E, Laflamme, R, Zurek, WH, Havel, TF, and Somaroo, SS (1998). Experimental quantum error correction. *Phys. Rev. Lett.*, 81, 2152–2155.

Cronin, AD, Schmiedmayer, J, and Pritchard, DE (2009). Optics and interferometry with atoms and molecules. *Rev. Mod. Phys.*, 81, 1051–1129.

Dahan, M, Levi, S, Luccardini, C, Rostaing, P, Riveau, B, and Triller, A (2003). Diffusion dynamics of glycine receptors revealed by single-quantum dot tracking. *Science*, 302, 442 – 445.

Dahlbom, M, Pullerits, T, Mukamel, S, and Sundstrom, V (2001). Exciton delocalization in the B850 light-harvesting complex: comparison of different measures. *J. Phys. Chem. B,* 105, 5515–5524.

De Vault, D and Chance, B (1966). Studies of Photosynthesis Using a Pulsed Laser I. Temperature Depen- dence of Cytochrome Oxidation Rate in Chromatium. Evidence for Tunneling. *Biophys. J.*, 6, 825–847.

Diosi, L (1989). Models for universal reduction of macroscopic quantum fluctuations. *Phys. Rev. A*, 40, 1165 – 1174.

Draguhn A, Traub RD, Schmitz D, Jefferys JGR Electrical coupling underlies high-frequency oscillations in the hippocampus in vitro. *Nature*, 1998, 394:189-192.

Dyson, GM (1938). The scientific basis of odour. *Chem. Ind.,* 57, 647–651.

Eccles J. *Evolution of the brain*, Routledge, Oxford, 1989

Eisert, J and Wiseman, H (2007). Quantum aspects of life, chapter *Nontrivial quantum effects in biology: A skeptical physicists' view*. World Scientific, Singapore.

Eisert, J, Wilkens, M, and Lewenstein, M (1999). Quantum games and quantum strategies. *Phys. Rev. Lett.*, 83, 3077–3080.

Engel, GS, Calhoun, TR, Read, EL, Ahn TY, Man?al, T, Cheng, YC, Blankenship, RE, and Fleming GR (2007). Evidence for wavelike energy transfer through quantum coherence in photosynthetic systems. *Nature*, 446, 782–786.

Forster, T (1948). Zwischenmolekulare energiewanderung und fluoreszenz. *Ann. Phys.* (Leipzig), ISSN:0003-3804, 2, 55–75.

Felker, PM, Lambert, WR, and Zewail, AH (1982). Picosecond excitation of jet-cooled pyrazine: magnetic field effects on the fluorescence decay and quantum beats. *Chem. Phys. Lett.,* 89, 309–314.

Gai, F, Hasson, KC, McDonald, JC, and Anfinrud, PA (1998). Chemical dynamics in proteins: The photoi- somerization of retinal in bacteriorhodopsin. *Science*, 279, 1886–1891.

Gardiner, C.W., *Handbook of stochastic methods for physics, chemistry and natural science*, Springer, 1983

Ghirardi, GC, Rimini, A, and Weber, T (1986). Unified dynamics for microscopic and macroscopic systems. *Phys. Rev. D,* 34, 470–491.

Glauber, RJ (2006). Nobel Lecture: One hundred years of light quanta. *Rev. Mod. Phys.,* 78(1267 - 1278).

Glickman, M, Wiseman, J, and Klinman, J (1994). Extremely large isotope effects in the soybean lipoxygenase-linoleic acid reaction. *J. Am. Chem. Soc.,* 116, 793–794.

Goldanskii, V (1979). Facts and hypotheses of molecular chemical tunnelling. *Nature*, 279, 109–115

Gray, H and Winkler, J (2003). Electron tunneling through proteins. *Quart. Rev. Biophys.*, 36, 341–372.

Hackermu¨ller, L, Hornberger, K, Brezger, B, Zeilinger, A, and Arndt, M (2004). Decoherence of matter waves by thermal emission of radiation. *Nature*, 427, 711–714.

Hackermu¨ller, L, Uttenthaler, S, Hornberger, K, Reiger, E, Brezger, B, Zeilinger, A, and Arndt, M (2003). Wave nature of biomolecules and fluorofullerenes. *Phys. Rev. Lett.*, 91(90408).

Hameroff S and Penrose R. Conscious events as orchestrated space time selections. N*euro Quantology* 2003; 1, 110-35

Hameroff, S and Penrose, R (1996). Orchestrated reduction of quantum coherence in brain microtubules: A model for consciousness. *Mathematics and computers in simulation*, 40, 453–480.

Harrow, AW, Hassidim, A, and Lloyd, S (2009). *Quantum algorithm for solving linear systems of equations.* arXiv:0811.3171v2.

Hecht, S, Shlaer, S, and Pirenne, M (1942). Energy, quanta and vision. *J. Gen. Physiol.,* 25, 819–840.

Hornberger, K, Uttenthaler, S, Brezger, B, Hackermu¨ller, L, Arndt, M, and Zeilinger, A (2003). Collisional decoherence observed in matter wave Interferometry. *Phys. Rev. Lett.*, 90(160401).

Johnsen, S and Lohmann, KJ (2008). Magnetoreception in animals. *Phys. Today*, 61, 29–35.

Jones, J and Mosca, M (1999). Approximate quantum counting on an NMR ensemble quantum computer. *Phys. Rev. Lett.*, 83, 1050–1053.

Jones, JA, Vedral, V, Ekert, A, and Castagnoli, G (2000). Geometric quantum computation using nuclear magnetic resonance. *Nature*, 403, 869–871.

Joos, E and Zeh, HD (1985). The emergence of classical properties through interaction with the environment. *Z. Phys. B.,* 59, 223–243.

Joos, E, Zeh, HD, Kiefer, C, Giulini, D, Kupsch, J, and Stamatescu, IO (2003). *Decoherence and the appearance of a classical world in quantum theory.* Springer, Berlin, 2nd edition.

Kaptein, R and Oosterhoff, JL (1969). Chemically induced dynamic nuclear polarization II: (Relation with anomalous ESR spectra). *Chem. Phys. Lett.,* 4, 195–197.

Kasprzak, J, Richard, M, Kundermann, S, Baas, A, Jeambrun, P, Keeling, JMJ, Marchetti, FM, Szymanska, MH, Andr´e, R, Staehli, JL, Savona, V, Littlewood, PB, Deveaud, B, and Dang, LS (2006). Bose-Einstein condensation of exciton polaritons. *Nature*, 443(7110), 409–414.

Keller, A and Vosshall, L (2004). A psychophysical test of the vibration theory of olfaction. *Nature Neuro- science*, 7, 337–338.

Koch C., Rapp M, Segev L. A brief histort of time (constant), *Celebral Cortex*, 1996, 6, 93-101

Kozlowski M, Marciak-Kozlowska J. Modified Schrodinger equation for particles with mass of the order of human neuron mass, *J Neuroquantology*, 8, 1-8, 2010

Kwiat, P, Mattle, K, Weinfurter, H, Zeilinger, A, Sergienko, A, and Shih, Y (1995). New high-intensity source of polarization-entangled photon pairs. *Phys. Rev. Lett.*, 75(24), 4337–4341.

Lauterbur, P (1973). Image formation by induced local interactions: examples employing nuclear magnetic resonance. *Nature*, 242, 190–191.

Levitan I. B. and Kaczmarek L. K. *The neuron: Cell and Molecular Biology*, New York, Oxford university Press, 1996

Levy-Leblond J M, Balibar F., *Quantic, Rudiments of quantum physics,* North Holland, 1990

Lidar, D, Chuang, I, and Whaley, K (1998). *Decoherence free subspaces for quantum computation*. quant-ph/9807004.

Lo¨wdin, PO (1963). Proton tunneling in DNA and its biological implocations. *Rev. Mod. Phys.,* 35, 724–732.

Longuet-Higgins, HC (1962). Quantum mechanics and biology. *Biophys J.*, 2, 207–215. Lounis, B and Orrit, M (2005). Single-photon sources. *Rep. Prog. Phys.,* 68, 1129–1179.

Maeda, K, Henbest, KB, Cintolesi, F, Kuprov, I, Rodgers, CT, Liddell, PA, Gust, D, Timmel, CR, andHore, PJ (2008). Chemical compass model of avian magnetoreception. *Nature*, 453, 387–390.

Marciak- Kozlowska J. Kozlowski M., *Thermal processes with attosecond laser pulses*, Springer, USA, 2006

Marcus, RA (1956). Theory of oxidation-reduction reactions involving electron transfer. *J. Chem. Phys.,* 24(5), 966–978.

Markham, D, Anders, J, Vedral, V, Murao, M, and Miyake, A (2008). Survival of entanglement in thermal states. *Eur. Phys. Lett.,* 81(40006).

Masgrau, L, Roujeinikova, A, Johannissen, L, Hothi, P, Basran, J, Ranaghan, K, Mulholland, A, Sutcliffe, M, Scrutton, N, and Leys, D (2006). Atomic description of an enzyme reaction dominated by proton tunneling. *Science*, 312, 237–241.

Matsuno, K (1999). Cell motility as an entangled quantum coherence. *BioSystems*, 51, 15–19.

McFadden, J (2000). *Quantum evolution: How physics' weirdest theory explains life's biggest mystery.* HarperCollins, New York.

Mohseni, M, Rebentrost, P, Lloyd, S, and Aspuru-Guzik, A (2008). Environment-assisted quantum walks in energy transfer of photosynthetic complexes. *J. Chem. Phys*, 129(174106).

Nielsen, MA and Chuang, IL (2000). *Quantum computation and quantum information.* Cambridge UniversityPress, Cambridge UK.

Nunez P L The brain wave equation: A model for EEG, *Mathematical Bioscience*, 1974, 21, 279-297,

Nunez P l, *Neocortical Dynamics and human EEG Rhythms*, Oxford University Press, 1995

Nunez P L, Srinivasan R., *Electric Fields of the Brain: The Neurophysics of the EEG*, 2nd Ed., Oxford University Press, London, 2006

Nunez, P. L *Brain, Mind, and the structure of reality*, Oxford University Press, 2010

Olaya-Castro, A, Lee, CF, Olsen, FF, and Johnson, NF (2008). Efficiency of energy transfer in a light- harvesting system under quantum coherence. *Phys. Rev. B,* 78(085115).

Penrose, R (1989). *The emperor's new mind: concerning computers, minds and the laws of physics.* Oxford University Press.

Penrose, R (1996). On gravity's role in quantum state reduction. *Gen. Rel. Grav.*, 28, 581–600.

Polson, RC and Vardeny, ZV (2004). Random lasing in human tissues. *Appl. Phys. Lett.*, 85, 1289–1291.

Prokhorenko, V, Nagy, A, Waschuk, S, Brown, L, Birge, R, and Miller, R (2006). Coherent control of retinal isomerization in bacteriorhodopsin. *Science*, 313, 1257–1261.

Rebentrost, P, Mohseni, M, Kassal, I, Lloyd, S, and Aspuru-Guzik, A (2009). Environment-assisted quantum transport. *New J. Phys.*, 11(033003).

Reiger, E, Hackermu¨ller, L, Berninger, M, and Arndt, M (2006). Exploration of gold nanoparticle beams for matter wave interferometry. *Opt. Comm.*, 264, 326–332.

Rieke, F and Baylor, D (1998). Single-photon detection by rod cells of the retina. *Rev. Mod. Phys.*, 70, 1027–1036.

Rieper, E, Gauger, E, Morton, JJL, Benjamin, SC, and Vedral, V (2009). *Quantum coherence and entan- glement in the avian compass.* arXiv:0906.3725.

Ritz, T, Adem, S, and Schulten, K (2000). A model for photoreceptor-based magnetoreception in birds.*Biophys. J.,* 78, 707–718.

Romero-Isart, O, Juan, ML, Quidant, R, and Cirac, JI (2009). *Towards quantum superposition of living organisms.* arXiv:0909.1469v1.

Sanchez-Mosteiro, G, Koopman, M, van Dijk, EMHP, Hernando, J, van Hulst, NF, and Garc´ıa-Para j´o, MF (2004). Photon antibunching proves emission from a single subunit in the autofluorescent protein DsRed. *Chem. Phys. Chem.,* 5, 1782–1785.

Schrödinger, E (1944). *What is life? The physical aspect of the living cell.* Cambridge Univ. Press.

Schulten, K, Swenberg, C, and Weller, A (1978). Biomagnetic sensory mechanism based on magnetic-field modulated coherent electron-spin motion. *Z. Phys. Chem.*, 111(1), 1–5.

Schuman W O, Uber die strahlunglosen Eingenschwingumgen einer leitenden Kugel, die von einer Luftschicht und einer Ionospharenhulle umgeben ist.*Z Naturforschung* 7a, 149-154, 1952

Sherson, J, Krauter, H, Olsson, R, Julsgaard, B, Hammerer, K, Cirac, I, and Polzik, E (2006). Quantum teleportation between light and matter. *Nature*, 443, 557–560.

Shor, P (1995). Scheme for reducing decoherence in quantum computer memory. *Phys. Rev. A*, 52, 2493–2496.

Sivozhelezov, V and Nicolini, C (2007). Prospects for octopus rhodopsin utilization in optical and quantum computation. *Phys. Part. Nucl. Lett.*, 4, 189–196.

Solov'yov, IA and Schulten, K (2009). Magnetoreception through cryptochrome may involve superoxide. *Biophys. J.,* 96, 4804–4813.

Tegmark, M (2000). The importance of quantum decoherence in brain processes. *Phys. Rev. E,* 61, 4194–4206.

Tronrud, D, Wen, J, Gay, L, Fenna, R, and Blankenship, RE (2009). *Unique bidentate ligation of a bacte- riochlorophyll found in an FMO antenna protein.* to be published, PDB ID: 3ENI.

Trost, J and Hornberger, K (2009). Hunds paradox and the collisional stabilization of chiral molecules. *Phys. Rev. Lett.,* 103(023202).

Turin, L (1996). A spectroscopic mechanism for primary olfactory reception. *Chem. Sens.*, 21(6), 773–791.

Turin, L (2002). A method for the calculation of odor character from molecular structure. *J. Theor. Biol.*, 216(3), 367–385.

Tuszyński J. A., Dixon J.M, *Biomedical Applications of Introductory Physics*, Wiley, 2002

van Grondelle, R and Novoderezhkin, V (2006). Energy transfer in photosynthesis: experimental insights and quantitative models. *Phys. Chem. Chem. Phys.*, 8(7), 793–807.

Vedral, V (2003). Entanglement hits the big time. *Nature*, 425, 28–29.

Vedral, V and Plenio, M (1998). Entanglement measures and purification procedures. *Phys. Rev. A*, 57(3), 1619–1633.

Watson, JDH and Crick, FHC (1953). Molecular structure of nucleic acids: A structure for deoxyribose nucleic acid. *Nature*, 171, 737–738.

Weaver, J, Vaughan, T, and Astumian, R (2000). Biological sensing of small field differences by magnetically sensitive chemical reactions. *Nature*, 405, 707–709.

Wiésniak, M, Vedral, V, and Brukner, Cˇ (2008). Heat capacity as an indicator of entanglement. *Phys. Rev. B*, 78(064108).

Wiltschko, R and Wiltschko, W (1995). *Magnetic orientation in animals.* Springer Berlin.

Wiltschko, R and Wiltschko, W (2006). Magnetoreception. *Bioessays*, 28, 157–168.

Winkler, J, Gray, H, Prytkova, T, Kurnikov, I, and Beratan, D (2005). *Bioelectronics, chapter Electron transfer through proteins, pages* 15–33. Wiley-VCH, Weinheim, Germany.

Woolf N.J. A possible role for cholinergic neurons of the basal forebrain and pontomesencephalon in consciousness, *Consciousness and Cognition.* 1997 6, 574-596,

Zarzo, M (2007). The sense of smell: molecular basis of odorant recognition. Biol Rev., 82, 455–479. Zurek, WH (1991). Decoherence and the transition from quantum to classical. *Phys. Today*, 44, 36–44.

Authors' Contact Information

Dr. Miroslaw Kozlowski
Warsaw University
Warsaw, Poland
miroslawkozlowski@aster.pl

Dr. Sultan Tarlaci
Department of Neurology, Associate Professor
Editor-In-Chief NeuroQuantology
Turkey

Index

B

C

D

E

F

G

H

K

L

M

N

O

P

Q

R

S

T